SOLVING CONUNDRUMS
IN
CLINICAL PSYCHIATRY

Presented with the compliments of

E. Merck Pharmaceuticals Ltd.

In memory of my parents,
and
to Efun and Lyn

SOLVING CONUNDRUMS IN CLINICAL PSYCHIATRY

A Guide to Viva Voce Examinations

by

Bankole A Johnson MB ChB MPhil MRCPsych
Department of Addictive Behaviour
Chilton Clinic
Warneford Hospital
Oxford
UK

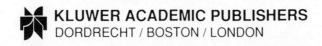
KLUWER ACADEMIC PUBLISHERS
DORDRECHT / BOSTON / LONDON

Distributors

for the United States and Canada: Kluwer Academic Publishers, PO Box 358, Accord Station, Hingham, MA 02018-0358, USA

for all other countries: Kluwer Academic Publishers Group, Distribution Center, PO Box 322, 3300 AH Dordrecht, The Netherlands

British Library Cataloguing in Publication Data

Johnson, B. A.
  Solving conundrums in clinical psychiatry.
  I. Title
  616.89

ISBN 0-79238-967-0

Copyright

Published in the United Kingdom by Kluwer Academic Publishers, PO Box 55, Lancaster, UK.

Kluwer Academic Publishers BV incorporates the publishing programmes of D. Reidel, Martinus Nijhoff, Dr W. Junk and MTP Press.

Lasertypeset by Martin Lister Publishing Services, Bolton-le-Sands, Carnforth, Lancs.

Printed and bound in Great Britain by Billing and Sons Ltd., Worcester

CONTENTS

19   School refusal, adolescent suicide, and   101
      non-accidental injury

20   Eating disorders   113

21   Panic disorder   121

22   Self-injurious behaviour   125

23   Complications of pharmacotherapy   129

24   Psychogenic regional pain   135

25   The irritating patient   139

26   Dementia and pseudodementia   142

27   Alcoholics and problem drinkers   152

28   Dynamic psychotherapy: assessment for treatment   161

29   Ethics and genetic counselling: Huntington's chorea   164

30   The mentally abnormal offender and the Mental   167
      Health Act

31   Paranoid state, morbid jealousy and folie à deux   177

32   Post-traumatic stress disorder and battle shock   184

      Main index   191

      Subject index   196

PREFACE

The idea for this book arose out of discussions with colleagues about issues of clinical management and the professorial unit formulation meetings at Oxford. Because the new format of the membership examination of the Royal College of Psychiatrists was based on clinical vignettes, it seemed logical to use similar questions to those posed in the examinations to devise management plans for conundrums in clinical practice. Although no book of this type could hope to be comprehensive, a wide range of clinical topics have been covered.

The style of the book is a verbatim response to clinical questions. For clarity, I have based my answers on what I would actually do which must, in part, reflect on my own training and experience. I am mindful, however, that clinicians (including examiners) often have strong views about treatment, particularly those of a psychological nature. I have, therefore, made every effort to give a balanced view of current clinical practice by having each question read by at least two colleagues. Additionally, I have expanded on special points of interest or controversial issues in the footnotes. Students would, however, be best advised to volunteer in an examination a type of psychological treatment with which he/she is familiar and can discuss in detail.

Throughout the book, I have, as far as possible, kept to a basic structure with clearly identifiable subheadings. Though it could be argued that, with experience, some of the questions could be answered with less restriction, this approach should help the candidate to think logically through even the most difficult questions and reduce the chance of important information being omitted.

Because most candidates prefer to revise topics by subject, a cross-index of the clinical vignettes by subject has been provided. Each question is followed by a list of up-to-date references and articles for further reading. For simplicity and consistency, I have chosen to reference one standard textbook of psychiatry (the *Oxford Textbook*) for background reading.

This book should be useful to candidates preparing for the final examination of the Royal College of Physicians or similar viva voce examinations in psychiatry. Furthermore, because some of the conundrums posed in this book are often met in clinical practice this *handbook* would also be a useful guide to all those involved in learning, debating and devising management plans in clinical psychiatry such as medical students, senior nurses, social workers, psychologists, and other mental health workers.

Bankole A Johnson
Oxford, 1991

ACKNOWLEDGEMENTS

I would like to express my profound gratitude to the following (in alphabetical order) for their helpful comments and advice:

Dr J Cutting
Dr R Fielsend
Dr K Fraser
Dr G Hibbert
Dr T Hope
Dr A James
Dr D Julier
Professor WA Lishman
Dr C Oppenheimer
Dr R Peveler
Dr M Sharpe
Dr C Ware

and

To my Tutors

I would also like to thank Mrs L Martyn, Miss P Hayward and Mrs A Gray for searching and obtaining original manuscripts.

EXAMINATION TECHNIQUES

Answering Viva Voce questions posed as clinical vignettes is essentially a test of communication and judgement. It would be worthwhile to remember that the examiner is likely to be as nervous as you – asking a silly question is, perhaps, more embarrassing than giving a silly answer – and that the questions may be based on problems which he/she may have faced (even in his/her personal life!). Therefore, do not be dogmatic, but try to approach the question in a logical fashion.

You may find the following tips helpful.

1. *Do not panic*: if your mind goes blank, it is best to start with an opening phrase which sets the tone of your answer – such openings have been extensively used in the book – and use the singular (e.g. I would ...).

2. *Use every scrap of information*: age, sex and occupation are frequently given, not to confuse, but to provide vital clues. Suggest treatments which are in keeping with the patient's clinical condition – for example, depressed elderly patients with heart disease should, preferably, be prescribed an antidepressant with a low risk of cardiotoxic side-effects and the dose should be built up slowly; conversely, it would not be sensible to recommend a large starting dose of an antidepressant which has been highly associated with cardiotoxicity. Special marks are often gained by tailoring your answer to the patient's circumstances – for example, there is a counselling and advice service for "sick doctors" and therefore suggesting a local voluntary group would not, in this case be appropriate. Furthermore, careful consideration should be given to weighing up the impact of the disorder on the patient's life. For instance, a patient's psychotic experiences may, in themselves, be manageable with appropriate medication on an outpatient basis but admission to hospital may still require serious consideration if the symptoms are associated with profound social disturbance, or there are certain factors in the community which are aggravating or maintaining the illness.

3. *Do not argue*: if your examiner disagrees with you, and tells you why, it is best to work constructively through the examiner's plan even if you have recently completed your PhD on the topic, or recently talked to the "world expert". It is exceedingly rare for an examiner to suggest a treatment plan that is unsuitable simply to trick you. If this occurs, the co-examiner would probably argue

your point, and may recommend to the college that he/she should be removed as an examiner.

4. *Be honest*: waffling simply irritates examiners. Try to construct a reasonable plan (e.g. biological, psychological and social), using the few facts you know, and if possible, suggest where the information you lack could be found.

5. *Watch the examiners*: if they are trying to move on, comply. If the question is asked again, this is probably a hint for you to think again. Accept prompts gracefully!

6. **Do not cross-question the examiner even if you think the question is silly or irrelevant**: for example, if you are asked about a man who developed panic attacks after visiting a male brothel, do not start off by questioning the legitimacy of such a brothel.[1]

7. *Communicate*: this comes with practice; therefore, organise mocks with your senior registrar or consultant. Record your mocks on a video, and play it back to chart your improvement. If you are having difficulty mastering this part of the examination, get yourself in to the right frame of mind beforehand – some candidates like to imagine they are being asked a similar question by their consultant on a ward round, or giving advice to another colleague by telephone.

8. *Do not, in your mind, carry out a post-mortem of your last question while answering the next*: if you have made a mess of your last question it would be better to concentrate harder on the next questions. If you do well with the others the chances are that you will be successful. You are, however, likely to feel worse if you allow a poor answer to mar the whole of your performance. Remember, keep your concentration!

9. *Think carefully about taking anxiolytics*: is this necessary? If you have a problem with exam nerves, enrol in an anxiety management class before the examination. Practice under simulated exam conditions also helps. When I sat the examination, I travelled to the exam centre by *Underground* with a colleague who had taken a β-blocker for the first time. Unfortunately for him, the escalator (to ground level) was out of order and we could not persuade or financially induce anyone to help carry him up over one hundred and fifty steps! If you feel compelled to take a β-blocker, make sure this has been rehearsed – fainting or developing marked hypotension or heart block could be counterproductive.

---

1 See question 14B.

10. *Appearance and behaviour*: much has been written about this elsewhere, but if in doubt, consult a senior colleague. Remember, you are presenting yourself as a future senior colleague, and it would be wise to appear suitable for the part.

GOOD LUCK!

CHAPTER 1

MUTISM AND STUPOR

QUESTION 1A

You are asked to see, on your psychiatric ward, a 20 year old man who has been brought in by the police. He was found mute and motionless by the side of the road. How would you assess him with a view to arriving at a differential diagnosis?

ANSWER 1A

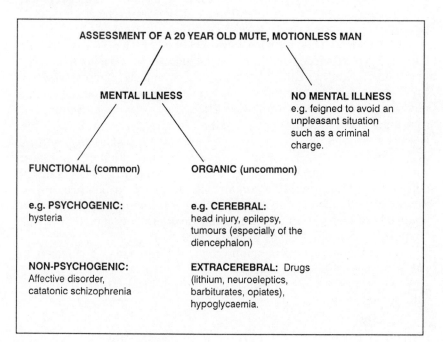

ASSESSMENT OF A 20 YEAR OLD MUTE, MOTIONLESS MAN

MENTAL ILLNESS

NO MENTAL ILLNESS
e.g. feigned to avoid an unpleasant situation such as a criminal charge.

FUNCTIONAL (common)

ORGANIC (uncommon)

e.g. PSYCHOGENIC:
hysteria

e.g. CEREBRAL:
head injury, epilepsy, tumours (especially of the diencephalon)

NON-PSYCHOGENIC:
Affective disorder, catatonic schizophrenia

EXTRACEREBRAL: Drugs (lithium, neuroleptics, barbiturates, opiates), hypoglycaemia.

ASSESSMENT

General opening/special features of the case

The purpose of my assessment would be to identify whether or not his *stupor* (mutism and motionless) was due to mental illness, and if so, its type (i.e. functional or organic).

Sources of history

I would need to observe and examine the patient, interview the policeman who brought him in, and record the accounts of any other available witnesses. I would see if he was carrying any personal information (e.g. medical alert or diary).

ASSESSMENT

History and mental state examination

Biological
I would use his personal details, if available, to contact his next of kin or friends (if appropriate), and to search for any relevant medical, psychiatric, social or forensic records.

I would observe his *appearance* and *behaviour*. I would like to know if he was: aware of his surroundings (i.e. if his eyes were open or shut, and if open, whether they followed events or objects. If shut, whether they responded to stimulation or resisted passive opening); malnourished, unkempt or unable to attend to matters of elimination; wearing the appropriate type of clothes for the time of year, or if his clothes were remarkable in any way; facially expressive (e.g. sad as in depression, or perplexed in response to hallucinations) or not, and whether this was maintained regardless of what was being said or done to him; maintaining a comfortable or awkward posture, and if the posture was fixed, whether he would resume a previous posture if moved or placed in an uncomfortable position; acting with "special" purpose or meaning (e.g. in response to delusions).

I would be suspicious of symptoms which appear to be inconsistent, exaggerated or paradoxical.

If he continued to be unresponsive, I would consider *abreaction* with sodium amytal.

Psychological
I would look for evidence of stressful *life events* and to be alert to *dissociative symptoms* and *secondary* gain (as in *hysteria*).

Social
I would look for social stressors, particularly those which may, preferably, be conveniently avoided, such as a criminal charge.

Physical examination

I would conduct a full physical and detailed neurological examination. At each stage, I would explain to the patient what I was about to do and why.

I would examine and quantify his level of consciousness (is he responding to: verbal commands, gentle pressure; painful stimuli, or nothing at all?) and muscle tone (i.e. is he relaxed or rigid, or is his tone increased by passive movement? Is there any evidence of *waxy flexibility* or *negativism*?). I would also look for evidence of: drug misuse (e.g. infections, needle tracks or enlarged lymph nodes); raised intracranial pressure; *diencephalic tumours*, and of upper brain stem disturbance (i.e. it would be important to test for papilloedema, equality and reactivity of the pupils, respiratory difficulty, long tract deficits, and conjugate reflex eye movements on passive head rotation.

I would take a blood specimen for a full blood count, electrolytes and blood sugar. An electroencephalogram may be necessary to distinguish between a functional or an organic cause of the stupor, and to diagnose epilepsy. I would carry out more specialised investigations such as a CAT scan, only if it is specifically indicated by the patient's clinical condition, or by the results of the investigations.

Differential diagnosis

See algorithm.

REFERENCES AND FURTHER READING

Gelder M, Gath D, Mayou R. *Oxford Textbook of Psychiatry* (second edition). Oxford: Oxford University Press, 1989; Chapter 11 p 363.

Johnson J. Stupor: its diagnosis and management. *British Journal of Hospital Medicine* 1982, 27: 530-32.

Joyston-Bechal MP. The clinical features and outcome of stupor. *British Journal of Psychiatry* 1966, 112: 967-81.

Lishman WA. *Organic Psychiatry* (second edition). Oxford: Blackwell, 1987.

QUESTION 1B

You are asked to see an 8 year old girl who is friendly and chatty at home, but refuses to speak at school.

How would you assess her? What is the differential diagnosis? How would you manage her?

ANSWER 1B

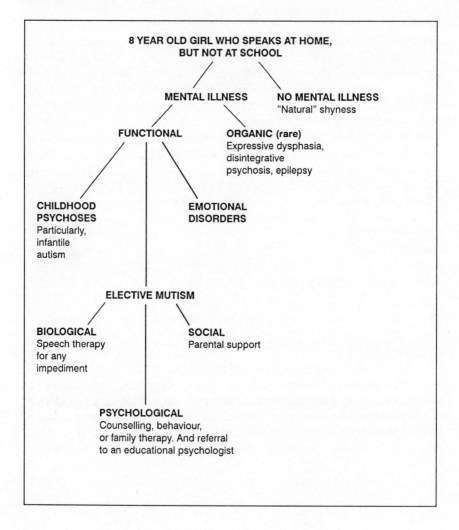

ASSESSMENT

General opening/special features of the case

The aim of my assessment would be to find out if her *mutism* was situation specific (i.e. elective), part of a more widespread functional or organic psychiatric disorder, or not due to mental disorder at all (i.e. "natural" shyness).

Sources of history

I would need to talk to the child's parents, her tutors, and the child herself.

History and mental state examination

Biological
I would take a full psychiatric and neurodevelopmental history. I would be particularly interested in the onset and progression of her symptoms (i.e. was there a provoking trauma? Is the mutism confined to school? Is the mutism associated with any other abnormalities of social interaction or communication for example, emotional aloofness?). I would also want to know if she has a history of: speech abnormality; any relevant medical conditions; compulsive traits; temper tantrums; negativistic or aggressive behaviour (especially in the home); elimination disorders (i.e. enuresis or encopresis); *dissociation* or *secondary gain*; psychotic[1] behaviour, or organic disorder (e.g. confusion, cognitive deterioration).

I would find out if there was a family history of mental illness or epilepsy.

Psychological
I would assess her personality (especially to know if she is "naturally" shy), and ascertain if there have been any significant *life events* or stresses such as parental separation. I would also look for evidence of *overprotection* in the home (particularly by her mother), and inquire more specifically about how she communicates at school (e.g. does she nod or shake her head? does she use grunts?). I would pay attention to any academic or cognitive difficulties which may be responsible for, or contribute to her symptoms. Psychometric testing may be necessary.

Social
I would wish to know if she has been able to form any social

---

1 Psychotic behaviour is often hard to identify accurately in children. It may take the form of bizarre behaviour, perplexity, or hallucinations. In any case, a detailed study of the child is needed by experienced observers.

relationships at school. for instance, is she liked, teased, or "scapegoated" by her peers?

Physical examination

I would carry out a detailed developmental and neurological examination. I would only proceed with more specialised tests such as an electroencephalogram or CT scan if it is clinically indicated.

Differential diagnosis

See algorithm.

MANAGEMENT

General opening/special features of the case

My management aims would be to treat the underlying cause of her mutism, and to get her settled at school.

Biological
If there was a speech abnormality causing embarrassment, and as a consequence, school avoidance, I would organise speech therapy.

Psychological
If the mutism was provoked by a specific trauma, counselling and behaviour therapy (i.e. a graded re-introduction to school and rewards for talking), would be appropriate. If the aetiology is less obvious, or the child is *overprotected* at home, I would opt for family therapy. A referral to the school's educational psychologist would also be appropriate.

Social
I would encourage her to join in activities at school, or at local clubs to improve her sociability.

REFERENCES & FURTHER READING

Cantwell PD, Baker L. Speech and language: Development and disorders. In: *Child and Adolescent Psychiatry, Modern Approaches*. Rutter M, Hersor L (editors). Oxford: Blackwell Scientific Publications, 1985 p. 531.

Fundudis T, Kolvin I, Garside R. *Speech Retarded and Deaf Children: Their Psychological Development*. London: Academic Press, 1979.

Gelder M, Gath D, Mayou R. *Oxford Textbook of Psychiatry* (second edition). Oxford: Oxford University Press, 1989: Chapter 20 p 805.

Wilkins R. A comparison of elective mutism and emotional disorders in children. *British Journal of Psychiatry* 1985; 146: 198-203.

CHAPTER 2
THE AGGRESSIVE PATIENT

QUESTION 2

You are bleeped by the nurse in charge of your ward to come immediately because a 22 year old well built male patient admitted overnight by your colleague, who was too tired to write up the notes, is assaulting a member of staff.

How would you manage this emergency?

What factors may have caused the violent behaviour?

ANSWER 2

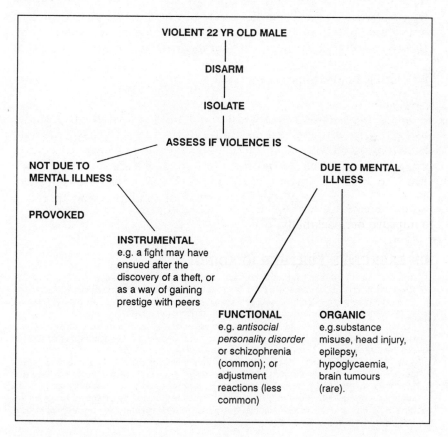

VIOLENT 22 YR OLD MALE

DISARM

ISOLATE

ASSESS IF VIOLENCE IS

NOT DUE TO MENTAL ILLNESS

DUE TO MENTAL ILLNESS

PROVOKED

INSTRUMENTAL
e.g. a fight may have ensued after the discovery of a theft, or as a way of gaining prestige with peers

FUNCTIONAL
e.g. *antisocial personality disorder* or schizophrenia (common); or adjustment reactions (less common)

ORGANIC
e.g.substance misuse, head injury, epilepsy, hypoglycaemia, brain tumours (rare).

MANAGEMENT

General opening/special features of the case

As I hurried to the ward, I would try to keep calm and, think about my plan of action.

Psychological

If I arrived on the ward and the patient was violent and armed, or the level of violence was clearly not containable by the staff, I would phone for the police to help disarm and isolate him. I would ensure that the staff and patients withdrew from the situation until the police had brought it under control. Any weapons taken from the patient would have to be disposed of in such a way (preferably by their removal from the premises) as to prevent its retrieval and re-use by the patient.

If unarmed, I would approach the patient (preferably in the company of a member of staff known to him) with sufficient staff so that if there was a confrontation, there would, in effect, be no contest. At first, I would try to *"talk down"* the patient in a calm, firm, but non-challenging voice, and use appropriate *"body language"*[1]. If this does not work, I would ask the staff to physically restrain[2] the patient and isolate him from the other patients in a side (or seclusion) room. Before instructing physical restraint to go ahead, I would ensure that all the staff participating in this knew exactly what their role would be during the restraining process.

Biological

If necessary, I would give medication to subdue the patient. I would, at first, offer any medication orally, but if this is refused, I would rapidly proceed with an intramuscular injection of either a sedative neuroleptic[3] (e.g. *chlorpromazine* 50–100 mg) or a short-acting barbiturate such as *sodium amytal* 200 mg. Because small doses of *benzodiazepines* may, paradoxically, increase disinhibition and therefore

---

1 Appropriate "body language" would include a relaxed stance and an attentive demeanour.

2 Nurses who have attended special courses in control and restraint may be particularly helpful. It is, however, worth remembering that if the aggression is due to mental illness and the ward staff are unable to contain it – this may be due to low staffing levels or not having enough nurses with the necessary skills – or if it becomes clear that the patient will require a long period of seclusion (>72 hours), consideration should be given to transferring the patient to a psychiatric intensive care unit.

3 While the clinical reports of a new sedative neuroleptic, *zuclopenthixol acetate*, which can be given daily as a single dose intramuscularly are encouraging, its use has not yet received widespread acceptance. Care must be taken to avoid severe extrapyramidal side-effects (particularly akathisia) when high doses of neuroleptics are used; they increase the patient's distress, and have been associated with increased violence (particularly in schizophrenia). β-Blockers may be used on their own or as an adjunct to neuroleptic treatment; often, however, their use is limited by profound bradycardia and hypotension. Lithium alone or in combination with carbamazepine are well known long-term treatments for aggression.

make the violence worse, I would avoid their use unless I was confident of being able to deliver a sufficient dose (*diazepam* 10–20 mg) intravenously. If the need for continuous medication arose, because of a recurrence of violence as the drug wore off, my preference would be to give the medication frequently (at half-hour to hourly intervals) and in small doses. In the event that this procedure is required for long periods (>24 hours), I would work out the total dose the patient received the day before, and if the violence was controlled, I would give the same total dose the next day, but at less frequent intervals. If the medication regime fails,[4] give *electroconvulsive* treatment if the violence was clearly motivated by psychosis. At all times, the patient's pulse, blood pressure, respiration and other vital signs – would be carefully monitored (at least hourly). If possible, I would try to carry out essential baseline investigations (full blood count, clinical chemistry and a urine drug screen).

I would review the case with the charge nurse at handover times and with a senior medical colleague; thus any management decisions taken would be jointly taken by the doctors and nurses.

Social
As soon as possible, I would *"debrief"* the staff and encourage the discussion of their fears and anxieties. I would hold a community group on the ward which, although not divulging any confidential details about the violent patient, would be aimed at reassuring the other patients that the ward was safe; this may also help with the re-introduction of the patient in to the ward environment after the violent episode.

ASSESSMENT

General opening/special features of the case

After the violent episode, I would find out if the violence had been due to provocation, mental illness, or an *instrumental motive*.

I would, of course, bear in mind that the motivation for violence may be complex (e.g. though the patient may be mentally ill, the violence itself may have been provoked by an argument).

Sources of history

I would need to obtain more information from: my colleague; the nurses who had been in contact with him (especially the nurse who had been assaulted by him); and interview reliable informants (i.e. friends or family), who could give an account of his personality, and events leading up to his admission. If he has a past psychiatric or

---

4 Medication regimes may fail to control the violence because the risk of toxicity may preclude the continued use of the drug or the administration of incremental doses.

relevant medical history, I would request the case notes and, if possible, speak to the consultants in whose care he had been.

I would interview the patient.

History and mental state examination

Biological

I would look for evidence of a formal mental illness: especially of an *affective disorder, adjustment reactions* or *schizophrenia.*

Psychological

I would look for a history of: antisocial behaviour in childhood; poor impulse control; threats to repeat violence; sadistic or paranoid fantasies; repeated episodes of violence; lack of provocation, regret or denial of violent acts; criminal activity; excessive alcohol intake or drug abuse; an antisocial personality with an inability to adjust appropriately to stressful situations.

Social

A history of chronic social difficulties and lack of support (particularly from the family) would not only be aetiologically important, but have implications for rehabilitation.

Physical examination

I would look for possible antecedents of the violent behaviour, and identify and treat any physical injuries he may have incurred. I would specifically look for evidence of alterations in his *level of consciousness, substance misuse* (e.g. needle tracks, enlarged lymph nodes infections) and signs of *raised intracranial pressure* (e.g. papilloedema). I would, as a baseline, perform a full blood count, electrolytes (including blood sugar), liver and thyroid function tests. More specialised investigations, such as an electroencephalogram to investigate epilepsy, would only be performed if it is clinically indicated.

Differential diagnosis – See algorithm.

REFERENCES AND FURTHER READING

Fottrell E. Violent behaviour by psychiatric patients. *British Journal of Hospital Medicine* (January) 1981: 28–37.

Gelder M, Gath D, Mayou R. *Oxford Textbook of Psychiatry* (second edition). Oxford: Oxford University Press, 1988: Chapter 22 p 895–6.

Haller RM, Deluty RH. Assaults on staff by psychiatric in-patients: a critical review. *British Journal of Psychiatry* 1988; 152: 174–9.

Perrin A. When crisis intervention gets physical. *Registered Nurse* 1989; 52(3): 36–40.

Schipperheijn JA, Dunne FJ. Managing violence in psychiatric hospitals. *British Medical Journal* 1991; 303: 71–2.

CHAPTER 3

POST-CONCUSSIONAL SYNDROME

QUESTION 3

A 50 year old businesswoman has been referred to you by her general practitioner because of a six month history of dizziness, headaches, irritability and general malaise after she tripped and fell over a loose stair carpet at work. She did not require any formal medical attention, and appeared to "come round" within a few minutes.

How would you assess her?

Would compensation by her employees reduce her symptoms?

ANSWER 3

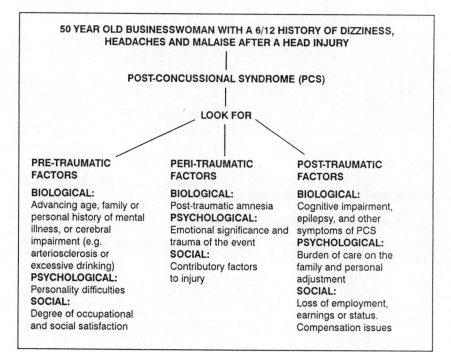

50 YEAR OLD BUSINESSWOMAN WITH A 6/12 HISTORY OF DIZZINESS, HEADACHES AND MALAISE AFTER A HEAD INJURY

|

POST-CONCUSSIONAL SYNDROME (PCS)

|

LOOK FOR

PRE-TRAUMATIC FACTORS	PERI-TRAUMATIC FACTORS	POST-TRAUMATIC FACTORS
BIOLOGICAL: Advancing age, family or personal history of mental illness, or cerebral impairment (e.g. arteriosclerosis or excessive drinking) **PSYCHOLOGICAL:** Personality difficulties **SOCIAL:** Degree of occupational and social satisfaction	**BIOLOGICAL:** Post-traumatic amnesia **PSYCHOLOGICAL:** Emotional significance and trauma of the event **SOCIAL:** Contributory factors to injury	**BIOLOGICAL:** Cognitive impairment, epilepsy, and other symptoms of PCS **PSYCHOLOGICAL:** Burden of care on the family and personal adjustment **SOCIAL:** Loss of employment, earnings or status. Compensation issues

ASSESSMENT

General opening/special features of the case

I would suspect that she had experienced a head injury during the fall due to her short loss of consciousness, and that her dizziness, headaches, irritability and general malaise were core symptoms of a *post-concussional syndrome (PCS)*.

The symptoms of PCS are both physiological and psychological in origin; thus, its assessment is dependent on knowing "the kind of brain that was injured", the extent of the brain injury, and her adaptation to it – that is, *pre, peri and post traumatic factors*.

Sources of history

I would interview the patient, her husband, and a reliable informant who witnessed the fall.

History and mental state examination

Biological
I would be interested in: **pre-traumatically**, a family or personal history of mental illness (especially of depression or anxiety), and any causes of cerebral impairment (e.g. excessive drinking or cerebral arteriosclerosis); **peri-traumatically**, the length of *post-traumatic amnesia* which is directly correlated with the severity of symptoms; and **post-traumatically**, any evidence of *intellectual or memory impairment* on cognitive testing, *epilepsy*, or *any other symptoms associated with PCS* such as depressed mood, emotional lability, insomnia, sensitivity to noise, decreased alcohol tolerance, and a **reduction in sexual interest**.

Psychological
I would look for: **pre-traumatically**, personality difficulties – there could be an excess of conflict situations, particularly in the marriage, an attitude of blaming previous unhappiness on the injury ("scapegoat motive"), or a tendency towards "neuroticism" which could impair the post-injury adjustment; **peri-traumatically**, the emotional significance and trauma of the event – for example, she could have a fear of "not waking from a coma", or there could have been the possibility of a catastrophic injury or loss of life (thus "shattering her myth of invincibility"); and **post-traumatically**, exploring the *burden of care* on her family, and how she herself has adjusted to her difficulties, would be important.

Social
I would ascertain: whether **pre-traumatically**, she was satisfied with her job and social life, look for recent *life events* (accidents are more

common in people in crisis) and note any contributory factors to the fall such as excessive drinking; **peri-traumatically**, the details of the accident – was she in a hurry? Was the stair case particularly dangerous? Was she distracted; who does she blame? Was there any resentment towards her employers? And **post-traumatically**, I would assess whether she had suffered any *loss of employment, earnings, or status*.

Compensation issues

Compensation and *litigation issues* would also be explored.

Traditionally, it was thought that the settlement of litigation concerning *PCS* was associated with a reduction in symptoms; in gainsay, more recent systematic investigation has failed to support this view.

REFERENCES AND FURTHER READING

Galasko CSB, Edwards DH. The causes of injuries requiring admission to hospital in the 1970's. *Injury* 1974; 6: 107–12.

Gelder M, Gath D, Mayou R. *Oxford Textbook of Psychiatry* (second edition). Oxford: Oxford University Press, 1989; chapter 11 p 369–72.

Kelly R. The post-traumatic syndrome. *Forensic Science* 1975; 6: 17–24.

McClelland RJ. Psychosocial sequelae of head injury – anatomy of a relationship. *British Journal of Psychiatry* 1988; 153: 141–6.

Miller HC. Accident neurosis. *British Medical Journal* 1961; i: 919–25 and 992–8.

Lishman WA. Physiogenesis and psychogenesis in the post-concussional syndrome. *British Journal of Psychiatry* 1988; 153: 460–9.

CHAPTER 4
SEIZURES AND PSEUDOSEIZURES

QUESTION 4

You have been asked to see a 25 year old foreign student who is due to return home in a month's time to be conscripted in to the Army. His general practitioner, who has no past medical history from his home country, and has not had time to examine him fully, believes his story of "fits" is suspicious.

How would you assess this situation?

ANSWER 4

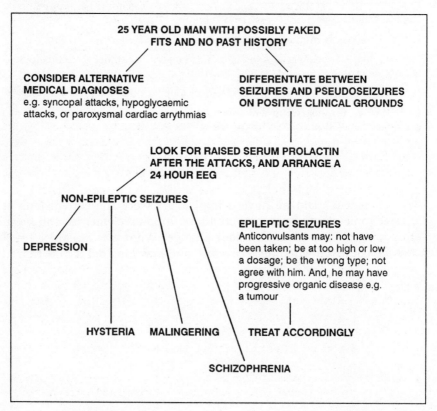

25 YEAR OLD MAN WITH POSSIBLY FAKED FITS AND NO PAST HISTORY

CONSIDER ALTERNATIVE MEDICAL DIAGNOSES
e.g. syncopal attacks, hypoglycaemic attacks, or paroxysmal cardiac arrythmias

DIFFERENTIATE BETWEEN SEIZURES AND PSEUDOSEIZURES ON POSITIVE CLINICAL GROUNDS

LOOK FOR RAISED SERUM PROLACTIN AFTER THE ATTACKS, AND ARRANGE A 24 HOUR EEG

NON-EPILEPTIC SEIZURES

DEPRESSION

EPILEPTIC SEIZURES
Anticonvulsants may: not have been taken; be at too high or low a dosage; be the wrong type; not agree with him. And, he may have progressive organic disease e.g. a tumour

HYSTERIA   **MALINGERING**   **TREAT ACCORDINGLY**

SCHIZOPHRENIA

ASSESSMENT

General opening/special features of the case

Non-epileptic seizures are commonest in people with epilepsy (which he could also have); thus the distinction between epileptic and non-epileptic seizures could be hard to make. And, because these "fits" could have been confused with some other organic condition such as a *syncopal attack, hypoglycaemic attack,* or *paroxysmal cardiac arrhythmia,* admission to hospital for a thorough investigation is frequently necessary.

Sources of history

I would interview witnesses to the seizures, and the patient himself.

History and mental state examination

Biological
The distinction between epileptic and non-epileptic seizures and pseudoseizures would be made on positive clinical grounds.

Firstly, I would look for a family or personal history of mental illness or epilepsy (his doctor overseas would have to be contacted) – a family or personal history of mental illness, attempted suicide, sexual maladjustment, and recent psycho-social stress are, comparatively, more commonly associated with non-epileptic seizures. He could also have a psychiatric disorder[1] (e.g. *depression*) presenting with non-epileptic seizures.

Next, I would obtain clinical details about the seizure: what was he doing before the attack? Was there any warning of the attack? Where and how frequently did the attacks take place? Was there always somebody around? Were the attacks dependent on his emotional state? What was his behaviour like during the attack? Did he lose consciousness? Did he have convulsions? Were the convulsions of classic tonic-clonic form, or were there unusual elements? Did he go limp or rigid? Did his skin colour change? What was his pulse rate? Was he confused when he recovered, and how long did it take him to recover? Does he have any memory of the event? *Strong clinical indicators of non-epileptic seizures* would include an insidious onset and very frequent attacks with a variable pattern, attacks which occurred in defined settings – usually in association with heightened emotionality – or accompanied by shouting, talking, struggling; there could also be a lack of tongue biting or an unusual pattern of injury.

---

1 Rarely, schizophrenia could also be associated with non-epileptic seizures; additionally, neuroleptic drugs used in its treatment could lower the seizure threshold and, thereby, produce epileptic seizures.

Thirdly, if I was unable to distinguish between the epileptic and non-epileptic seizures, solely on clinical grounds, I would perform corroborative investigations – the *serum prolactin* is raised for up to twenty minutes compared with baseline levels, following a generalised epileptic seizure (usually to levels >1000 IU/ml), and *24 hour ambulatory electroencephalographic monitoring* would provide the best opportunity to detect pathognomic electrical activity. Computerised axial tomography could also provide evidence to support a diagnosis of epilepsy such as cortical atrophy or changes suggestive of Ammon's horn sclerosis.

Fourthly, if he had a pre-existing diagnosis of epilepsy, before the development of the suspicious "fits", I would consider the possibility that its control had deteriorated – for example, the *anticonvulsants* might: not have been taken; have been the wrong choice for his type of epilepsy; have been prescribed at too high or too low a dosage (check serum levels); be producing an idiosyncratic reaction. And, there could be progression of an underlying organic condition such as a *tumour*.

Psychological
Fifthly, I would assess his personality and details of psychosocial situation for evidence of secondary gain (i.e. hysteria).

Social
Sixthly, I would examine whether the stress[2] returning home to join the army could have lead him to manufacture the non-epileptic seizures.

And, I would be interested in the reactions of his friends and family and their level of support to his seizures.

Physical examination

I would undertake a thorough physical (to identify his injuries) and neurological examination (especially for evidence of *raised intracranial pressure*).

REFERENCES AND FURTHER READING

Hopkins A. *Epilepsy: the facts*. Oxford: Oxford University Press, 1981.

Lishman WA. *Organic Psychiatry* (second edition). Oxford: Blackwell, 1987.

Scott DF. Too many fits. *British Journal of Hospital Medicine* (December) 1984: 306–11.

Trimble M. Pseudoseizures. *British Journal of Hospital Medicine* (April) 1983: 326–33.

---

2 Stressful life events can increase the frequency of organic epileptic seizures.

CHAPTER 5

TREATING DRUG ADDICTION

QUESTION 5A

A 40 year old Army Officer who tells you he is an intravenous user of heroin, and who says he wants to give up, using heroin alone, is sent to you by his general practitioner. The officer also tells you he is to be posted abroad in a week and, therefore, wants something done immediately.
    What will you say?
    How will you manage this problem?

ANSWER 5A

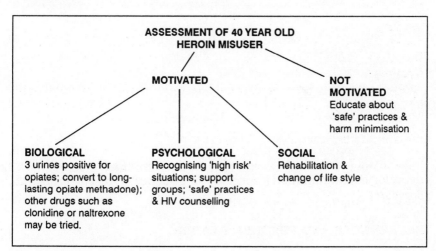

ASSESSMENT

General opening/special features of the case

Management is dependent on assessment. There are, however, three salient features to this case. They are: (a) It is not yet established whether or not he genuinely misuses drugs; (b) the demand for heroin is suspicious, and may, therefore, be motivated by other factors such as financial gain; and (c) his imminent posting abroad.

Sources of history

Although I would like to corroborate his history of drug misuse with either a member of his family or a reliable informant, it is not always possible to get the patient's permission to do this. If the family is made available however, I would like to know about the effect of his drug taking on the family – particular attention would be paid to changes in his: behaviour (e.g. increased social withdrawal); social circle (to include other drug misusers); medical well-being (e.g. recurrent infections) and increasing financial problems, which may be associated with illegal activities to raise money to buy drugs.

History and mental state examination

Biological
I would like to take a full history of substance (alcohol and drug) misuse and concentrate on: the types and amounts of substances misused; pattern of substance dependence (including periods of abstinence); how and with whom the drugs were injected and if needles or syringes were shared. I would find out what he knew about 'safe' sex and HIV infection. I would look carefully for any evidence of associated mental illness.

Psychological
I would assess: his willingness to stop or reduce his intake using the *motivational interview* technique and a *decision matrix*[1]; personality (**chasm: c** – character, **h** – habits, **a** – attitudes, **s** – standards, **m** – predominant mood); and identify situations which put him at '*high risk*' of taking drugs (e.g. excessive alcohol consumption). I would inquire about recent life events and any continuing stressors.

Social
I would evaluate his coping skills and deficits.

In addition to determining the impact of drug taking on his personal life, I would ask him whether his posting could be postponed to allow him to receive immediate treatment or whether he would be willing to take up treatment either abroad or on his return home.

Physical examination

I would examine him thoroughly for both local (e.g. venous throm-

---

1 A *decision matrix* is a simple two-part table compiled by the patient listing the pros and cons of drug use, which is systematically reviewed by a counsellor using problem solving techniques.

bosis, abscesses, damaged arteries) and general (e.g. hepatitis, septi-caemia) effects of drug use. I would take blood for a full blood count, liver function test, hepatitis and syphilis screen. No HIV testing will be carried out without prior counselling and the full consent of the patient. A urine sample will be taken for a drug screen – the patient would be advised that he will need to supply urine samples on the following two consecutive days, the results of which must be positive for the allegedly misused drug, before treatment can begin.

MANAGEMENT

General opening/special features of the case

I would inform the patient that only specially licensed doctors in the United Kingdom may legally prescribe heroin to addicts (in practice, this iᴗ usually only done in exceptional circumstances such as 'high dose' heroin dependence). I will also tell him that all doctors in the United Kingdom must (under the Misuse of Drugs Notification of Supply to Addicts Regulations 1973) notify the Chief Medical Officer of the names of people addicted to heroin and related compounds.

Regardless of whether or not the patient is willing or able to remain in this country, or for any reason does not wish to accept further medical help, he should be given advice on practising 'safe sex', harm reduction (e.g. how to obtain both sterile needles and syringes and to inject properly) and offered Human Immunodeficiency Virus (HIV) counselling.

Biological
A firm contract would be agreed by both the patient and myself before any withdrawal programme begins. If the heroin use is severe, or complicated by other factors (e.g. polydrug use or mental illness), I would consider admission to a specialist centre.

The total daily dose of heroin would be converted to the equivalent dose of methadone (1 mg heroin $\equiv$ 1 mg methadone). I would ad-minister the total daily dosage in four divided doses. As a rough time guide, in-patient withdrawal regimes take between 10–21 days; while for outpatients, a period of six to eight weeks is reasonable. Other drug treatments such as clonidine and naltrexone are possibilities, and I would introduce these treatments only on the advice of a specialist.

Psychological
I would recommend to the patient that he attend a therapeutic group (these are usually run by local voluntary organisations) for support and relapse prevention work. I would work with him, on an individual basis, on how to avoid 'high risk' situations.

Social

I would advise him that in order to remain drug free he will need a period of rehabilitation. Thus, he might need to avoid: friends in the 'drug scene'; move home; change to a more stable or less stressful occupation and if his dependence has been particularly severe or chaotic, he may need a period of time in a therapeutic community.

REFERENCES AND FURTHER READING

Drummond C, Edwards G A, Glanz A et al. Rethinking drug policies in the context of acquired immunodeficiency by syndrome. *Bulletin of Narcotics* 1987, 39(2): 29–35.

Gelder M, Gath D, Mayou R. *Oxford Textbook of Psychiatry* (2nd edition). Oxford: Oxford University Press, 1989: Chapter 2 p 46–47 and Chapter 4 p 537–47.

Greenwood J. Creating a new drug service in Edinburgh. *British Medical Journal* 1990; 300: 587–9.

Trenes J W, O'Brien C P. The opioids: abuse liability and treatments for dependence. *Advances in Alcohol and Substance Abuse* 1990; 9(1–2): 27–45.

Van Bilsen HP, Von Emst AJ. Heroin addiction and motivational milieu therapy. *International Journal of the Addictions* 1986; 21(6): 707–713.

QUESTION 5B

A 70 year old female patient is referred to your outpatient clinic. She has been receiving 1mg of lorazepam at night for the last 15 years for disturbed sleep after a bereavement. She tells you she wants to come off as she recently watched a television programme which told her the drug was "poisonous". She is extremely worried and still has 'trouble sleeping'. She has a past history of depression which was treated with antidepressants and ECT 20 years ago.

(a) How will you manage the problem?

(b) What will you say when counselling her about her fears?

ANSWER 5B

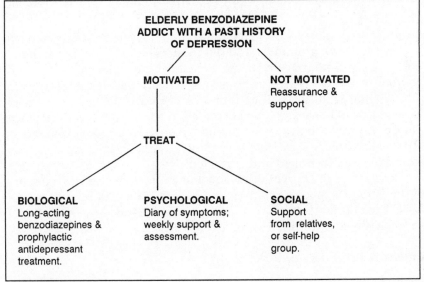

ASSESSMENT

General opening/special features of the case

Management is dependent on assessment. The salient points of the assessment are whether an elderly woman who has been receiving a short-acting *benzodiazepine* for many years, with no clear benefit, but with no adverse effects either, should be weaned off benzodiazepines? And, what are the chances of this weaning off process being successful, and what is the risk of a relapse of the depression?

Sources of history

Informants are particularly useful in the assessment of elderly patients. Thus, I would interview the patient first and subsequently, corroborate the history with the account of a close relative (especially her husband if possible), or any person who had either accompanied her to the clinic or been involved in her case.

History and mental state examination

Biological
I would be interested in an accurate picture of the patient's sleep, appetite and weight, the nature and course of any past or current history of anxiety or depression, and inquiring about a family psychiatric history of depression. I would ensure there was no current evidence of an abnormal grief reaction and find out whether the patient had any history of forgetfulness and formally test her cognitive function. I would also look for any personality change or disinhibition.

Psychological
I would openly discuss the fears and anxieties the patient experienced during the TV programme. I would be mindful that the TV programme may, simply, have triggered off adverse memories from either her past or from recent life events or stressors; it would also be important to discuss non-medical such as financial problems as well as medical issues. I would assess her motivation[2] to come off benzodiazepines after a thorough (but without the use of medical jargon) explanation of the withdrawal syndrome – negative experiences or expectations will have to be identified and corrected.

The success of any withdrawal regime is dependent on the support of the patient's spouse, relatives and friends. Thus, as far as practicable, I would educate them too – a printed hand out, or a simple self-help book, if available, would be provided.

Physical examination

I would look for any evidence of gait disturbance (e.g. bruising due to falls) and test the patient's co-ordination. I would test a urine sample, if readily available, for glucose (benzodiazepines can aggravate diabetes).

MANAGEMENT

General opening/special features of the case

The priority would be only to proceed with a withdrawal regime in this patient if she is highly motivated or there are important medical contraindications such as cognitive impairment. If the decision is made not to proceed with a withdrawal regime, simple reassurance

---

2 Motivation can be assessed using the motivational interview technique (cross reference question 5A).

(benzodiazepines can not strictly be classified as poisons since endogenous ligands probably exist) and support is usually sufficient.

Biological
In view of her past history of a depressive illness, and especially if there is also a family history of depression, it would be prudent to provide the patient with prophylactic antidepressant treatment during the withdrawal period. An anxiolytic antidepressant of proven *cardiac safety* in the elderly such as *lofepramine* (between 70 and 140 mg/day) is advisable; it may also help to ameliorate some of the rebound symptoms.

To reduce the severity of rebound symptoms, the short-acting benzodiazepine she is receiving (*lorazepam 1 mg/day*) should be changed to a longer-acting compound (e.g. *diazepam* 10 mg/day). Since the majority of patients on long-term benzodiazepines do not experience intolerable rebound symptoms with a brisk withdrawal regime, I would opt for this strategy. Other adjunctive therapies such as beta-receptor adrenoreceptor antagonists are of limited value. *Clonidine* is ineffective.

I would like to see the patient weekly and aim to reduce the dose of diazepam by half each week or until withdrawal symptoms dictate a more gradual dose reduction. I would aim for a 6–8 week withdrawal period, but would be prepared to be flexible if necessary.

Psychological
Since formal psychological help is not often helpful or practicable, I would offer regular pragmatic but non-directional advice. I would encourage the patient to keep a diary of her symptoms and discuss them with her at our meetings; a watchful eye would be kept for the emergence of psychological symptoms wrongly attributed by the patient to the withdrawal syndrome.

Social
I would encourage and monitor the support the patient receives from her spouse, relatives, or friends. If this is insufficient, I would refer her to a local self-help group or day centre.

REFERENCES AND FURTHER READING

Gelder M, Gath D, Mayou R. eds. *Oxford Textbook of Psychiatry* (2nd edition). Oxford: Oxford University Press, 1989; Chapter 17, 639–641.

Hallstram C. The uses and abuses of benzodiazepines. *British Journal of Hospital Medicine* 1989; 41: 115.

Lader M H. Benzodiazepine withdrawal In: Glass I ed. *International Handbook of the Addictions*. London: Routledge, 1991.

Tyrer R, Murphy S. The place of benzodiazepines in psychiatric practice. *British Journal of Psychiatry* 1987; 151: 719–23.

CHAPTER 6

AGORAPHOBIA

QUESTION 6

You have been asked by a general practitioner to see a 25 year old housewife with a one month history of episodes of panic when she goes shopping. She has become almost housebound due to her avoidance of crowded places, and has to rely on her husband to do the shopping.

What is the most likely diagnosis?

Give a brief outline of your management.

ANSWER 6

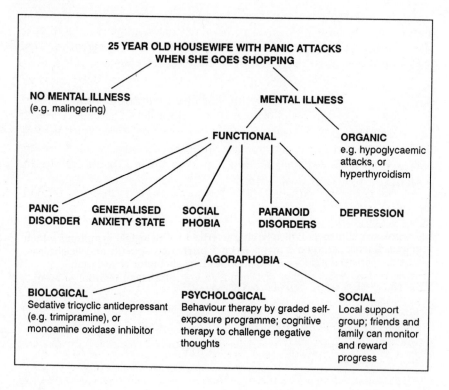

DIAGNOSIS

The most likely diagnosis is *agoraphobia*.

ASSESSMENT

General opening/special features of the case

Management would be dependent on assessment, the purpose of which would be to identify any concurrent mental illness such as depression or dangerous coping mechanisms, and to determine the degree of *psycho-social disability*.

Sources of history

I would interview her at home with her husband, separately at first, and then together.

Biological
I would: *firstly*, look for a family or personal history of phobias or depression;

secondly, explore the nature, onset and progression of her symptoms to identify any associated psychopathology which could include *panic attacks, depression,*[1] depersonalization or obsessions, and to exclude other functional disorders – for examples, a generalised anxiety state, panic disorder,[2] social phobia (usually, there is widespread anxiety in all social settings since adolescence or earlier), or a paranoid illness (persecutory delusions could be present) – or an organic condition (e.g. hypoglycaemic attacks, hyperthyroidism, or drug withdrawal);

thirdly, look for any dangerous coping mechanisms such as alcohol or drug misuse (particularly of benzodiazepines);

---

1 A depressive illness is typically characterized by biological symptoms which include diurnal variation of mood, sleep disturbance, appetite and weight loss, fatigue, decreased libido, constipation and psychomotor retardation.

2 In the revised third edition of Diagnostic and Statistical Manual of Mental Disorders (DSM IIIR), published by the American Psychiatric Association, Washington DC (1989), panic disorder is divided into two categories: those with or without agoraphobia. Panic disorder is characterized by one or more panic attacks (discrete episodes of intense fear or discomfort) that were (1) unexpected, i.e. did not occur immediately before or on exposure to a situation that almost always caused anxiety, and (2) not triggered by situations in which the person was the focus of others' attention. Four or more attacks must have occurred within a four week period or one or more attacks have been followed by at least a month of persistent fear of having another attack. The attacks must not be due to an organic condition – mitral valve prolapse may be an associated condition but does not preclude a diagnosis of panic disorder.

Psychological
fourthly, be interested in any *negative cognitions* (particularly fears about fainting, loss of control, or anticipation of further panic attacks); *fifthly*, inquire about contributory *life events*;[3]

Social
sixthly, determine the *impact of her illness* on interpersonal (including marital[4]) relationships, and look for any evidence of *abnormal illness behaviour* (e.g. malingering or factitious disorder).

MANAGEMENT

General opening/special features of the case

Worsening agoraphobia symptoms are often associated with a depressive illness.

A sedative tricyclic antidepressant (e.g. *dothiepin*) would be used to treat a concurrent depressive illness and relieve anxiety. And in common with monoamine oxidase inhibitors, tricyclic antidepressants reduce the severity of agoraphobic symptoms by an unknown mechanism; an antidepressant would, however, not be used on its own to treat agoraphobia due to the high risk of relapse when the drug was stopped.

Benzodiazepines, for symptomatic relief of anxiety, would be avoided because of their potential to cause dependence.

Psychological
I would provide the patient with guidance on how to carry out a self-exposure programme to the feared situation – she would have to remain in this situation for up to two hours (i.e. until her anxiety[5] habituates). These exposure exercises would be carried out daily, recorded in a homework diary, and reviewed with me at predetermined intervals. Additionally, cognitive therapy could be used to challenge persistent negative thoughts.

Social
Attendance at a local support group[6] would be encouraged, and friends and family could be asked to monitor and reward progress.

A *problem-solving* approach would be used to address interpersonal or marital conflicts.

---

3 Life events are not commonly associated with agoraphobia.
4 Although serious marital problems are infrequent in agoraphobia, there are often minor conflicts about roles and power sharing.
5 Other anxiety reducing measures such as relaxation therapy are seldom needed.
6 Information on support groups can be obtained from a lay group in Bath, England (C Bonham-Christie, European Association of Behaviour Therapy, Paris, 1990).

REFERENCES AND FURTHER READING

Gelder M, Gath D, Mayou R. *Oxford Textbook of Psychiatry* (second edition). Oxford: Oxford University Press, 1989; chapter 7 p 186–90.

Marks IM. Phobias and related anxiety disorders. *British Medical Journal* 1991; 302: 1037–8.

Marks IM. *Living with Fear*. New York: McGraw Hill, 1978.

CHAPTER 7

DEPRESSION AND PUERPERAL DEPRESSION

QUESTION 7A

A 31 year old solicitor who gave birth four months ago to her first baby has been unable to return to work. The pregnancy was unplanned. The baby was premature and had to be nursed in an incubator for a month. Her husband has complained to their general practitioner that she has been depressed, always tired and irritable since the birth of the child. Also, he says she is not coping with looking after the baby. The general practitioner has requested your help.

What would your management be?

ANSWER 7A

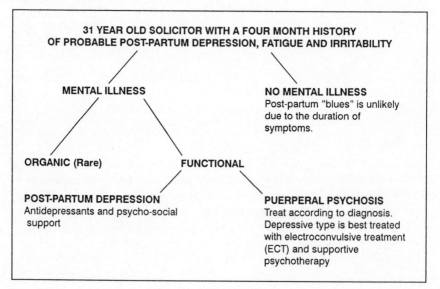

ASSESSMENT

General opening/special features of the case

Management is dependent on assessment.
I would find out if her symptoms were the result of a mental disorder (particularly depression) and assess its severity. I would also assess the risk of the patient harming herself or the child.

Sources of history

I would interview the patient and her husband – separately at first, and subsequently, together.

History and mental state examination

Biological
I would look for a past personal or family history of mental illness (especially of puerperal depression or psychosis), and carefully explore the onset and progression of her symptoms.[1] I would specifically look for evidence of a depressive illness, and for psychotic symptoms such as hallucinations and delusions which could contain "messages" or ideas that the child was deformed, evil, or needed to be killed to spare it from future suffering. I would assess suicide risk[2] and I would attempt to make a distinction between *psychotic phenomena*, and *obsessional ruminations* about harming the child (which are usually the product of low self-esteem and are seldom acted upon).

I would look for evidence of organic mental disorder by testing her cognitive function.

Psychological
I would find out if the patient had: ambivalent feelings about having the baby and about the responsibility of motherhood; a lack of "*bonding*" with her child due to their enforced separation; a stable relationship with her own mother (e.g. what was her own experience of childhood like? were there any separations? can her mother be counted on to help?); any conflicts between her role as a woman and as a professional; a satisfactory relationship with her husband (e.g. is he supportive, unduly passive, or over-dominant?); experienced any recent *life events*.

---

1 *Puerperal psychosis* is characterised by: an early and rapid onset of symptoms (usually within the first fortnight following childbirth); and a prodromal phase lasting about two days of insomnia, irritability, food refusal and depression, lability of mood, elation or grandiosity, and confusion. There is a slow progression of anxiety, fatigue, restlessness, sleep difficulty and loss of libido in *post-partum depression*.
2 Assessment of suicide risk: cross reference question 17A.

Social

I would look for changes in her circumstances which may have increased her vulnerability, such as an alteration in financial or social status, and attend to any practical problems.

MANAGEMENT

General opening/special features of the case

This patient is most likely to have a *post-partum depression.*

I would try to treat the depression at home, and to use as much of her own and her family's resources as possible. If admission is necessary, I would maintain contact between mother and child, preferably on a mother and baby unit, to foster *bonding.*

If there was no mental illness, I would offer support and encouragement.

Biological

I would prescribe a tricyclic antidepressant. Because tricyclic antidepressants are excreted in breast milk, it would be prudent to consider a transfer from breast to bottle feeding. I would consider ECT if the depression is severe, or associated with psychotic symptoms.

Psychological

I would provide the patient and her husband with *support* and encouragement. Specific or refractory interpersonal problems would be approached using a *problem-solving* technique.

Social

Practical advice could be of considerable help in many instances.

REFERENCES AND FURTHER READING

Dean C, Kendall RE. The symptomatology of puerperal illness. *British Journal of Psychiatry* 1981; 139: 128–33.

Gelder, M, Gath D, Mayou R. *Oxford Textbook of Psychiatry* (second edition). Oxford: Oxford University Press: Chapter 12 p 466–470.

Paykel ES, Emms EM, Fletcher J et al. Life events and support in puerperal depression. *British Journal of Psychiatry* 1980; 136: 339–46.

Pitt B. 'Atypical' depression following childbirth. *British Journal of Psychiatry* 1968; 114: 1325–35.

QUESTION 7B

On your ward, there is a 65 year old widow who was diagnosed as having a major depressive illness for which she has been receiving 200 mg nocte of amitriptyline for the last three months without any improvement. Her eldest daughter, who is a professor of sociology, believes electroconvulsive therapy (ECT) is barbaric. How would you manage this situation?

ANSWER 7B

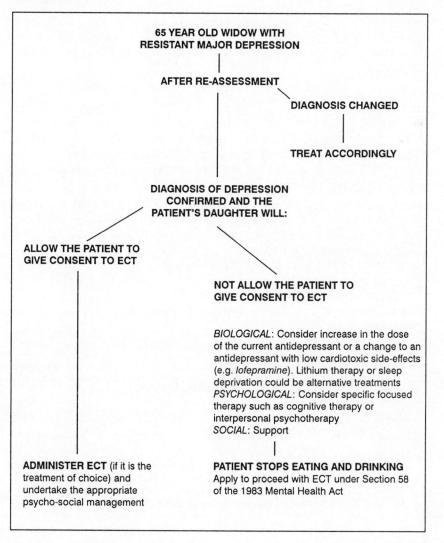

65 YEAR OLD WIDOW WITH RESISTANT MAJOR DEPRESSION

AFTER RE-ASSESSMENT

DIAGNOSIS CHANGED

TREAT ACCORDINGLY

DIAGNOSIS OF DEPRESSION CONFIRMED AND THE PATIENT'S DAUGHTER WILL:

ALLOW THE PATIENT TO GIVE CONSENT TO ECT

NOT ALLOW THE PATIENT TO GIVE CONSENT TO ECT

BIOLOGICAL: Consider increase in the dose of the current antidepressant or a change to an antidepressant with low cardiotoxic side-effects (e.g. *lofepramine*). Lithium therapy or sleep deprivation could be alternative treatments
PSYCHOLOGICAL: Consider specific focused therapy such as cognitive therapy or interpersonal psychotherapy
SOCIAL: Support

ADMINISTER ECT (if it is the treatment of choice) and undertake the appropriate psycho-social management

PATIENT STOPS EATING AND DRINKING
Apply to proceed with ECT under Section 58 of the 1983 Mental Health Act

ASSESSMENT

General opening/special features of the case

Management would be dependent on assessment.

The aim of my assessment would be to re-assess: the diagnosis of depression and its severity; and the risk of suicide[2], or of a dangerous deterioration in her health.

Sources of history

Any medical or psychiatric notes.

I would also interview the patient, any other reliable informants (including relevant ward staff), and plan to see her daughter on her own.

History and mental state examination

Biological

I would look for any medical or psychiatric disorders that could be mimicking or contributing to her symptoms of depression. I would find out if she has been taking her antidepressants regularly (by inquiring about the presence of anticholinergic side-effects), or any medication (e.g. antihypertensives such as alpha-methyldopa) which could have made the depression resistant to treatment. If she has a past history of depression, I would be interested in its onset, progression, and response to treatment.

I would make a careful note of all her depressive[3] symptoms, particularly those that predict a good response to ECT,[4] and assess her *suicide risk*.

I would test her cognitive function to exclude an organic disorder (especially dementia).

Psychological

I would pay attention to any interpersonal, interfamilial, or intrapsychic (e.g. an unresolved grief reaction) conflicts that could be maintaining the depression.

Social

If I thought that ECT was the treatment of choice, I would ascertain:

---

3 Once the diagnosis of depression has been made on clinical grounds, the depressive symptoms can be charted on a standardised rating scale (e.g. *Hamilton Depression Scale*: after Hamilton M, *Journal of Neurology and Psychiatry* 1960; 23: 56–62) on which serial measurements of change can be quantified.

4 Predictors of a good response to ECT in the elderly, in addition to the biological symptoms of depression are agitation, marked guilt, and a premorbid obsessional personality.

how much her daughter knew about ECT, and the likelihood of changing her mind about it by a non-confrontational and educational (about the risk/benefit ratio) interview; if other members of the family were of the same opinion as the daughter and if not, could they persuade her to change her mind?

Physical examination

I would carry out a full medical and neurological examination, and review the investigations.[5] It would be essential to, at first, look for common treatable conditions such as anaemia or infections, and relatively less common but important disorders like *hypothyroidism*, *Parkinson's*, or *metastatic* disease.

MANAGEMENT

General opening/special features of the case

It would be essential to monitor her depressive[3] symptoms, and to ensure that she is on weight, sleep, calorie, and fluid intake chart.

Biological
If she stopped eating and drinking and could not give *informed consent*, I would apply to proceed with ECT[6] under Section 58[7] of the Mental Health Act 1983. Otherwise it would be good clinical practice to try to work with her daughter by considering other treatment strategies after a full consideration and explanation of their relative risks. For examples: with regular cardiac monitoring[8] an increase in the dose of antidepressant (amitriptyline) could be considered or a change to an antidepressant with low cardiotoxic side-effects (e.g. *lofepramine*). *Lithium therapy*, could be used as an adjunct to anti-depressant treatment. *Sleep deprivation* could also be a useful treatment.

---

5 Essential baseline investigations include a full blood count, thyroid function test, liver function test, urine culture, urea and electrolytes, serum calcium, liver function test, erythrocyte sedimentation rate and chest X-ray.
6 Unilateral ECT is preferable (to reduce memory impairment), and almost as effective as bilateral.
7 *Section 58 of the Mental Health Act 1983* refers to treatment requiring consent or a second opinion and includes ECT or pharmacotherapy for longer than three months. An independent doctor must confirm in writing that the patient is unable to understand the nature, purpose and likely effects of treatment, but that, having considered the likelihood of its improving or preventing the deterioration of the patient's condition, the treatment should be administered.
8 Cardiac monitoring includes regular measurements of pulse, blood pressure, and electro-encephalographic recordings.

Psychological
In addition to biological treatments, I would consider specific focused therapy such as *cognitive therapy* or *interpersonal psychotherapy*.[9]

Social
An often overlooked, but frequently effective, management strategy would be to support the patient, and make her as comfortable as possible while waiting patiently for a remission (rather than opt for potentially risky pharmacological treatments).

REFERENCES AND FURTHER READING

Benbow S.M. The role of electroconvulsive therapy in the Treatment of old age depression. *British Journal of Psychiatry* 1989; 155: 147–52.

Gelder M. Psychological treatment for depressive disorder. *British Medical Journal* 1989; 300: 1087–8

Gelder M., Gath D., Mayou R. *Oxford Textbook of Psychiatry* (second edition). Oxford: Oxford University Press 1989; Chapter 8 p. 262–4.

Jacoby R. Depression in the elderly. *British Journal of Hospital Medicine* (January) 1081: 40–7.

Leonard B.E. Biochemical aspects of therapy resistant depressions. *British Journal of Psychiatry* 1988; 152: 453-9.

---

9 Interpersonal psychotherapy plus antidepressants is better than antidepressants alone in treating resistant depression.

CHAPTER 8
MÜNCHAUSEN'S SYNDROME

QUESTION 8

You have been asked to see a 25 year old man in casualty who claims to have taken 200 × 500 mg tablets of paracetamol four hours ago (his paracetamol level was zero when tested). He also says that his father was a famous brain surgeon who was shot dead by the relative of a patient who died in his care a year ago and he has, therefore, been left a rich man. He says that he has recently bought a new Ferrari and that his girl friend gave birth to triplets two days ago. He is convinced that the Iraqis have invaded America and admits to hearing the voice of his dead father telling him to kill himself. He says he sees visions, and is able to read other people's thoughts and project his own. Subjectively, he does not appear to be distressed by his thoughts. There is also no evidence of thought disorder and he looks well nourished and reasonably dressed.

What are your thoughts?

How would you assess him?

ANSWER 8

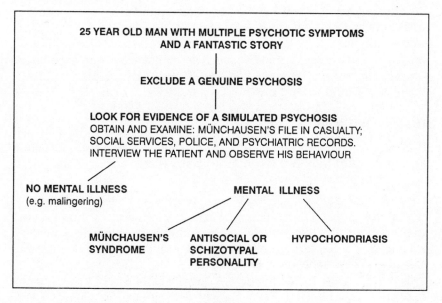

ASSESSMENT

General opening/special features of the case

The large number of psychotic symptoms in the absence of any objective evidence of distress, the negative paracetamol level, and the incredible story (reminiscent of *pseudologia fantastica*) would suggest that he was *simulating a psychosis*.

The purpose of the assessment would be to substantiate my suspicion that he had a *factitious disorder*, to exclude the unlikely possibility of a psychotic illness such as schizophrenia, and to consider the other possibilities.

The factitious disorders to consider would be *malingering* or *Münchausen's syndrome*. Alternatives include antisocial (which should be evident from his past history) or schizotypal personality disorder (characterised by magical thinking, ideas of reference, and derealization), or hypochondriasis (unlikely due to his age, and because such patients do not willingly volunteer symptoms or submit themselves to treatment). Drug abusers may also invent stories to gain access to hospital.

Sources of history

I would interview: the patient and obtain relevant personal details; any members of staff who could describe his behaviour in Casualty or who had any prior knowledge of him; and look for any reliable informants. Because he could refuse to volunteer personal details or give fictitious information, I would note his physical characteristics. What was known about him would, subsequently, be cross-checked with information kept in the *Münchausen's file* in Casualty. If there was no match in the file, and my suspicions remained strong, I would attempt to locate him using the *social service register*, and the police's *"missing or wanted" persons file*. And if there was a local psychiatric hospital, I would extend my inquiries to include them.

History and mental state examination

If all of the inquiries above prove to be inconclusive, I would play it safe and admit him to the ward for observation.

Biological
I would painstakingly look for inconsistencies and irregularities in his psychiatric and medical history. Particular attention would be paid to his *appearance and behaviour* – was there any evidence of neglect; was he distressed at any time by his experiences; was he eating and sleeping well; was he interacting normally with other patients; was he selective in what he told different members of staff? – and to the *quality of his symptoms*. For instance, were the "voices": in or outside

his head; heard through his ears; male or female; in the second or third person; conveying any distinct messages; affected by his state of arousal or by the time of day?

It would also be essential for me to look for traumatic childhood experiences (especially those which resulted in multiple or prolonged periods of hospitalization, and as a consequence, separation from his parents), and to determine how far he is prepared to go to sustain his account of illness (malingerers usually give up their symptoms when asked to comply with painful, uncomfortable, or potentially hazardous treatments).

Psychological
I would look carefully for any recent or anticipated life events – for example, his symptoms could be motivated by *secondary gain* (suggesting Münchausen's syndrome) such as an attempt to deliberately avoid an unpleasant situation (e.g. imprisonment).

Social
I would be interested in the reaction of members of staff and of the other patients to him – did they: think he was ill; like him; feel sorry for him or want to help him; find him too demanding or irritating; think his symptoms were manufactured, and what evidence did they have of this?

REFERENCES AND FURTHER READING

Asher R. Munchausen's Syndrome. *Lancet*, 1951; i: 339–41.

Gelder M, Gath D, Mayou R. *Oxford Textbook of Psychiatry* (second edition). Oxford, Oxford University Press, 1989: Chapter 12 p 418–9.

King BH, Ford CV. Pseudologia fantastica. *Acta Psychiatrica Scandinavica*, 1988; 77: 1–6.

Raspe RE. *The Singular Travels, Campaigns and Adventures of Baron Münchausen*. London: Cresset Press, 1948.

CHAPTER 9

NEUROLEPTIC-RESISTANT MANIA

QUESTION 9

You have been asked to see a 30 year old man on the ward who was admitted with a diagnosis of mania by virtue of overactivity, irritability, restlessness, persecutory (including grandiose delusions), second and third person auditory hallucinations and flights of ideas of four weeks duration. During that time, he has received between 0.9 g and 1.2 g of chlorpromazine daily with no change in his mental state.

What would your management be?

ANSWER 9

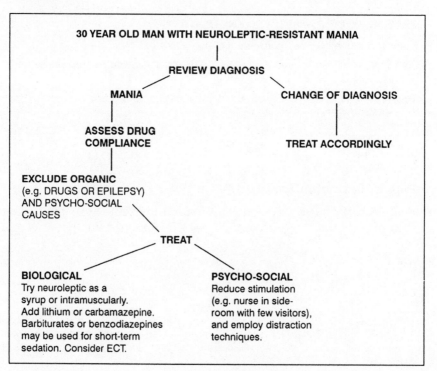

ASSESSMENT

General opening/special features of the case

The successful management of *neuroleptic-resistant mania*, essential to prevent exhaustion, and to aid recovery, would be dependent on a three part assessment: a review of the diagnosis, checking compliance to medication, and exploring relevant psycho-social factors.

Sources of history

I would interview the patient, and obtain information from reliable informants and key members of staff.

History and mental state examination

Biological
I would look for evidence: that the diagnosis should have been of a more chronic disorder such as *schizophrenia* – up to 25% of schizophrenic patients show manic symptoms and *vice versa*; of an organic explanation – for instance, an *elevation in his liver enzymes* would, proportionally, reduce the drug serum concentration – or cause[1] for his illness (e.g. drugs of abuse such as cannabis, which mimic manic symptoms, could have been supplied to him on the ward by a relative, other patients, or even a member of staff; or, he could be *epileptic*); of *non-compliance to medication* (he may have been observed to discard or refuse to take his medication, or there may be an absence of extrapyramidal side-effects).

Psycho-social
Psycho-social factors either on or off the ward could be maintaining the illness. For examples, unresolved family conflicts could manifest as an association between the deterioration in his clinical condition and family visits, or he could be overstimulated or frustrated at being confined to the ward.

Physical examination

I would carry out a physical examination to exclude organic causes of mania such as hyperthyroidism and drug abuse (the possibility of human immunodeficiency virus infection would also be borne in mind). I would ensure that his full blood count, urea and electrolytes, liver and thyroid function test, and syphilis serology had been checked. Additionally, I would undertake a urine drug screen.

---

1 For a description of clinical signs on cognitive testing which would suggest an organic cause see Krauthamner C, Klerman GL. Secondary mania: manic syndromes associated with antecedent physical illness or drugs. *Archives of General Psychiatry* 1978; 35: 1333–9.

Electroencephalographic studies would be done if there was clinical suspicion of epilepsy.

MANAGEMENT

General opening/special features of the case

For an uncomplicated case of neuroleptic-resistant mania, I would adopt the following plan.

Biological

Firstly, I would not increase his dose of chlorpromazine (indeed, a small reduction could be warranted) or change to another neuroleptic[2] Alternatively, his tablets would be changed to a syrup, and its administration would be supervised for at least an hour afterwards, to prevent self-induced vomiting.

Secondly, if the change to the syrup was ineffective, I would administer the medication intramuscularly in small divided doses.

Thirdly, for short-term behavioural control, a barbiturate or benzodiazepine (e.g. sodium amytal or clonazepam respectively) could be added. I would be careful not to produce *paradoxical disinhibition* by giving too low a dose.

Fourthly, for more long-term control of symptoms, *lithium, carbamazepine, sodium valproate* or *clonidine* could be used within their therapeutic range.

Fifthly, if aforementioned pharmacological strategies were unsuccessful, I would, having obtained the necessary consent, administer *bilateral electroconvulsive treatment* (on alternate days, and up to a maximum of 12, until his symptoms had been brought under control.

Psycho-social

Sixthly, I would *reduce his level of stimulation* by nursing him in a side-room, restricting his visitors, and observing him as unobtrusively as possible.

Seventhly, I would encourage the use of distraction techniques.

REFERENCES AND FURTHER READING

Chalmers J. Mania: what if neuroleptics don't work? In: *Dilemmas and Difficulties in the Management of Psychiatric Patients*, Hawton K and Cowen P (editors). Oxford: Oxford University Press, 1990.

---

2 Rarely, some patients respond to very high doses of neuroleptics; more usually, however, this leads to clinical deterioration. Changing neuroleptics, often to haloperidol, is also of doubtful value, and there may be the added complication of not being able to safely start lithium treatment. The use of high potency preparations at elevated dosages is largely based on clinical impression, and the increased risk of severe extrapyramidal side-effects such as tardive dyskinesia or neuroleptic malignant syndrome should be borne in mind.

Gelder M, Gath D, Mayou R. *Oxford Textbook of Psychiatry* (second edition). Oxford: Oxford University Press, 1989; chapter 8, 257–8 and 265–7.

Small JG, Small IF, Milstein V et al. Manic symptoms: an indication for bilateral ECT. *Biological Psychiatry* 1985; 20: 125–34.

CHAPTER 10
THE "SICK DOCTOR"

QUESTION 10

You are asked by a consultant anaesthetist to see his colleague who is performing poorly at work. The theatre nurses have complained that in the mornings he is tremulous and there is always the smell of alcohol on his breath. At lunchtime he insists on going to the pub for a drink. At social gatherings he is often drunk and argumentative with his wife. How would you manage this problem?

ANSWER 10

See algorithm on next page

ASSESSMENT

General opening/special features of the case

This is the case of the "*sick doctor*" whose excessive alcohol consumption is impairing his professional judgement. Usually, in order to manage a clinical problem, I would first need to make a full assessment of its onset, nature and progression. This, however, is a special situation because the referral has taken place without the consent of the person concerned (i.e. the "sick doctor"). Thus, all I could offer would be advice as to what management options are.

MANAGEMENT

General opening/special features of the case

The answer to two questions govern management. They are: is the "sick doctor" willing to accept help?; and, how risky is it for him/her to continue to treat patients?

Advice
If the "*sick doctor*" refuses to seek help and is putting patients' health at risk, the referring doctor has no option but to bring the matter to the attention of the hospital managers who representing the Health Authority. If the hospital managers are also unable to persuade the "sick doctor" to seek help the case is referred to the *General Medical Council (GMC)*. This type of referral to the GMC is initially dealt with

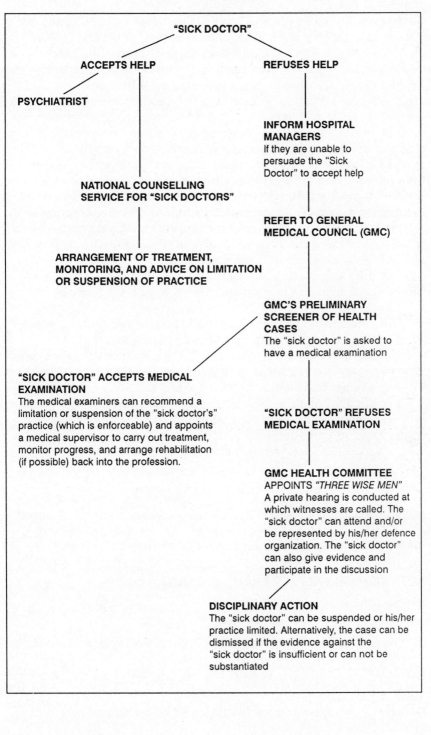

"SICK DOCTOR"

ACCEPTS HELP

REFUSES HELP

PSYCHIATRIST

INFORM HOSPITAL MANAGERS
If they are unable to persuade the "Sick Doctor" to accept help

NATIONAL COUNSELLING SERVICE FOR "SICK DOCTORS"

REFER TO GENERAL MEDICAL COUNCIL (GMC)

ARRANGEMENT OF TREATMENT, MONITORING, AND ADVICE ON LIMITATION OR SUSPENSION OF PRACTICE

GMC'S PRELIMINARY SCREENER OF HEALTH CASES
The "sick doctor" is asked to have a medical examination

"SICK DOCTOR" ACCEPTS MEDICAL EXAMINATION
The medical examiners can recommend a limitation or suspension of the "sick doctor's" practice (which is enforceable) and appoints a medical supervisor to carry out treatment, monitor progress, and arrange rehabilitation (if possible) back into the profession.

"SICK DOCTOR" REFUSES MEDICAL EXAMINATION

GMC HEALTH COMMITTEE
APPOINTS *"THREE WISE MEN"*
A private hearing is conducted at which witnesses are called. The "sick doctor" can attend and/or be represented by his/her defence organization. The "sick doctor" can also give evidence and participate in the discussion

DISCIPLINARY ACTION
The "sick doctor" can be suspended or his/her practice limited. Alternatively, the case can be dismissed if the evidence against the "sick doctor" is insufficient or can not be substantiated

by the *Preliminary Screener of health cases* who would invite the "sick doctor" to receive a medical examination by a specialist in his/her own locality, and then to accept the examiner's recommendations for any necessary medical treatment and limitation or suspension of his/her practice. Subsequent treatment is provided by medical supervisors who make progress reports to the GMC's screener. If the sick doctor refuses to accept the GMC's request for a medical examination, or fails to comply with the management plan put forward by the medical examiners or supervisors, the case is brought before the GMC's Health Committee. Subsequently, the Chairman of the Health Committee appoints a panel of three doctors (*"Three Wise Men"*) to conduct a private hearing. The "sick doctor" is invited to attend this hearing (and/or can be represented by his/her defence organization), during which he/she may answer questions, and participate in the discussion of evidence. Witnesses are usually called. The *"Three Wise Men"* have the power to take whatever disciplinary action is necessary against the "sick doctor". Alternatively, the case can be dismissed if the evidence against the "sick doctor" is insufficient or can not be substantiated.

If the "sick doctor" agrees to accept help (it is frequently necessary to ask other colleagues, a close relative or the spouse to assist with persuading the "sick doctor" to seek help), he/she can self-refer, or be referred by a colleague to a psychiatrist of his/her choice or the *National Counselling Service for "sick doctors"* (NCS). The NCS operates a telephone hotline (071–580–3160), and has a network of advisors and counsellors in all specialities throughout the country. It is highly confidential and provides help outside the "sick doctor's" own district.

The Counselling service is only advisory and can not compel the "sick doctor" to accept treatment, or take disciplinary action against him/her.

Rehabilitation of the "sick doctor", by either the GMC or the NCS, is co-ordinated by medical supervisors, and can include a change to a less stressful discipline of medicine or a limitation on his/her practice.

REFERENCES AND FURTHER READING

Kilpatrick R. Helping the "sick doctor": the work of the GMC's Health Committee. *Journal of the Royal Society of Medicine* 1988; 81: 436–37.

Pilowski L, O'Sullivan G. Mental illness in doctors. *British Medical Journal* 1989; 298: 269–70.

Rawnsley K. "Sick doctors". *Journal of the Royal Society of Medicine* 1986; 79: 440–41.

Rucinski J. Mentally ill doctors. *British Journal of Hospital Medicine* February 1985: 90–4.

CHAPTER 11

ASSESSMENT OF RELAPSE AND OF CHRONIC SCHIZOPHRENIA

QUESTION 11A

A 19 year old male in-patient who was successfully treated with neuroleptics for schizophrenia, and who has been asymptomatic for several months is allowed home on weekend leave for the first time. He returns after the weekend in an agitated state, and says he believes he is being persecuted by the devil. Indeed, he says he has been hearing the devil call his name. How would you assess him? What are the likely causes?

ANSWER 11A

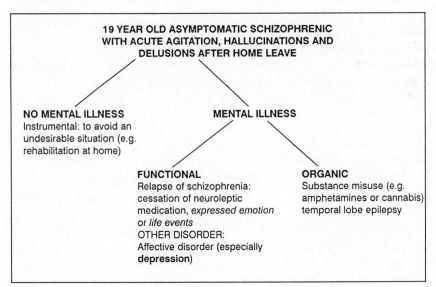

ASSESSMENT

General opening/special features of the case

Due to the acute development of psychotic symptoms (second person auditory hallucinations and paranoid delusions) on his return home and, because he had not been home for several months, even though he was asymptomatic, I would suspect that factors at home may be associated with his symptoms.

Although second person auditory hallucinations may occur in schizophrenia, they are more characteristic of affective disorder.

Sources of history

I would like to interview the patient, and, separately, any members of his family or friends who were at home with him during the weekend. And I would review his psychiatric notes.

History and mental state examination

Biological
I would obtain details of the nature, onset and progression of his symptoms, and compare his current symptoms with those on which the diagnosis of schizophrenia was based. Affective disorder, especially *depression*, would be important to exclude as it may, initially, have been indistinguishable from either the *negative symptoms of schizophrenia* (e.g. blunting of affect) or the *tardive effect* of neuroleptic drugs.

I would find out if he had been taking his prescribed drugs (i.e. neuroleptic medication) regularly while at home, a reduction or absence of extrapyramidal side-effects would be suspicious. Additionally, I would ascertain whether he had the motive, means, or opportunity to misuse illicit substances such as amphetamines or cannabis).

I would test his cognitive function, primarily for any evidence of an *acute confusional state*, or any other organic disorder which may have been overlooked (e.g. *temporal lobe epilepsy*).

Psychological
I would carefully evaluate the level of *expressed emotion* (i.e. critical comments. hostility, or overinvolvement) in the home environment, and inquire about any recent *life events*.

Social
I would ascertain whether, at home, he had coped satisfactorily with daily living, the stress of re-learning basic tasks can be frustrating, and whether he was given the appropriate level of responsibility and stimulation; *overstimulation* could have provoked the relapse.

I would look for any evidence of *over-dependence* on the ward environment.

Physical examination

I would conduct a physical and neurological examination, and perform a full blood count, urea and electrolytes and a urine drug screen.

Differential diagnosis

See algorithm.

REFERENCES AND FURTHER READING

Brown GM, Birley JLT. Crisis and life change at the onset of schizophrenia. *Journal of Health and Social Behaviour* 1968; 9: 203–24.

Brown GM, Monck EM, Carstairs GM et al. Influence of family life on the cause of schizophrenic illness. *British Journal of Preventative and Social Medicine* 1962; 16: 55–68.

Connell PH. *Amphetamine Psychosis*. Maudsley Monograph No. 5. London: Oxford University Press, 1958.

Flor-Henry P. Psychosis and temporal lobe epilepsy. *Epilepsia* 1969; 10: 363–95.

Gelder M, Gath D, Mayou R. *Oxford Textbook of Psychiatry* (second edition). Oxford: Oxford University Press, 1989; chapter 9 p 282, 312–314.

Johnson BA. Psychopharmacological effects of cannabis. *British Journal of Hospital Medicine* 1990; 43: 114-22.

QUESTION 11B

You have on your ward a 26 year old man admitted two months ago with a diagnosis of schizophrenia characterized by third person auditory hallucinations, persecutory delusions and thought disorder. He has, however, made no clinical improvement despite large doses of neuroleptic medication. At present, he is receiving two neuroleptics (chlorpromazine 1.2 g/day, droperidol 20 mg/day as required), an anticholinergic (procyclidine 30 mg/day), and an antidepressant (amitriptyline 25 mg nocte) which was prescribed by his general practitioner for anxiety six months ago.

How would you manage him?

ANSWER 11B

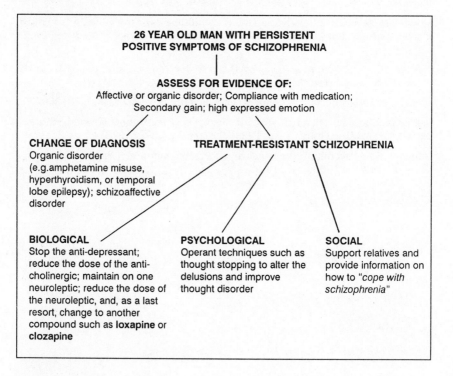

ASSESSMENT

General opening/special features of the case

Management is dependent on assessment, the aim of which would be to investigate the reasons for the *treatment-resistant schizophrenia*.

Sources of history

I would interview the patient, his key nurse, and a close friend or relative.

History and mental state examination

Biological
I would: *firstly*, ascertain whether he has been taking his medication (while *extrapyramidal signs* such as rigidity or tremor on clinical examination would suggest a certain degree of compliance, confirmation of full compliance would, however, require *serial measurements of serum prolactin*).

Secondly, review the diagnosis, particularly for evidence of *affective* or *organic disorder* (e.g. amphetamine misuse, temporal lobe epilepsy,[1] or *human immunodeficiency virus (HIV)*[2] *infection*), by exploring the family and personal history, and carrying out a mental state examination.

Psychological
thirdly, look for any proof of *secondary gain* – atypical, exaggerated, or more prominent symptoms in the presence of others would be suspicious;

Social
fourthly; consider the possibility that his illness was being maintained by *high expressed emotion (EE)* – attention would be paid to interpersonal conflicts with other patients, staff, or visiting relatives.

Physical examination

I would look for evidence of: drug misuse – for examples, infections, scars, or needle tracks – and carry out regular *random urine drug screens*; *unexplained falls or injuries*; and review the results of his investigations. Thyroid and liver function tests would be repeated.

MANAGEMENT

General opening/special features of the case

There are six steps to managing *treatment-resistant schizophrenia*.

Biological
Firstly, I would stop the antidepressant, maintain him on one neuro-

---

1 Temporal lobe epilepsy, particularly of the left lobe, is associated with increased risk of schizophrenia (see Flor-Henry P. Epilepsy and psychopathology. In: *Recent Advances in Clinical Psychiatry* Volume 2, Granville-Grossman K (editor).

2 HIV infection is an increasingly common cause of major psychiatric disorder.

leptic[3] (*chlorpromazine*), and reduce the possibility of anticholinergic toxicity by bringing its dose back into the therapeutic range (up to 20 mg daily).

Secondly, if compliance was a problem, the medication would be prescribed as a syrup, and its administration supervised for an hour afterwards (to prevent self-induced vomiting), or given intramuscularly.[4]

Thirdly, while some patients benefit from high doses of neuroleptics, the majority do not; I would, therefore, consider a small reduction in the dose of chlorpromazine.

Fourthly, if all the above strategies fail to improve his condition, I would consider a trial with a drug of reported benefit in treatment-resistant schizophrenia (e.g. *loxapine* or *clozapine*);[5] although some clinicians would also consider electroconvulsive treatment, the case for its use remains unconvincing.

Psychological
Fifthly, if pharmacological treatments produce no improvement, I would attempt to modify his delusions and thought disorder using *operant techniques* such as thought stopping. The intensity of the auditory hallucinations could be reduced by getting him to wear an *ear plug*, and teaching him *distraction* and *relaxation techniques*.

Social
Sixthly, if he remained chronically disabled by his symptoms, I would continue to provide support, and educate his family about how to "*cope with schizophrenia*".[6]

---

3 The practice of taking a neuroleptic drug to the limit of its therapeutic range and then adding another increases rather than decreases the risk of toxicity, and should be avoided.

4 Neuroleptics induce liver enzymes; thus, an elevation to several times its baseline value, would, by a similar proportion, reduce the serum drug concentration. Because intramuscular injection of the neuroleptic would avoid the first pass metabolism of the liver, administration by this route would give rise to comparatively higher serum concentrations than would have been achieved if the same dose had been given orally.

5 Cross reference: footnotes of question 23A for the precautions to follow with *clozapine treatment*.

6 A useful book for relatives on how to cope with schizophrenia is: *Living and Working with Schizophrenia*, Seeman MV, Littmann SK, Plummer E et al (editors), published by the Open University Press, Oxfordshire (1982).

REFERENCES AND FURTHER READING

Bebbington PE, Kuipers L. Non-physical treatment of the psychoses. *British Medical Bulletin* 1987; 43: 704–17.

Connell PH. *Amphetamine Psychosis*. Maudsley Monograph No 5. London: Oxford University Press, 1958.

Gelder M, Gath D, Mayou R. *Oxford Textbook of Psychiatry* (second edition). Oxford: Oxford University Press, 1989; chapter 9 p 270–2.

Johnstone EC. Chronic schizophrenia: can one do anything about persistent symptoms? And, Taylor PJ. Schizophrenia and ECT: a case for a change in prescription? In: *Dilemmas and Difficulties in the Management of Psychiatric Patients*, Hawton K and Cowen P. (editors). Oxford: Oxford University Press, 1990.

Kane J, Honigfeld G, Singer J et al. Clozapine for the treatment-resistant schizophrenic. *Archives of General Psychiatry* 1988; 45: 789–96.

QUESTION 11C

You have been asked to attend a ward round on the long-stay ward by your consultant at which a 55 year old woman with a 30 year old history of schizophrenia is discussed. She has had no acute symptoms for the last fifteen years, and over that period, has been receiving 40 mg of fluphenazine decanoate intramuscularly every month. The staff on the ward are pessimistic about rehabilitating her in to the community because she is difficult to motivate, withdrawn, neglectful of her personal hygiene, and lacking in appropriate speech. She has no living relatives.

What would you say if your consultant asks you to briefly outline your management plan at the ward round?

ANSWER 11C

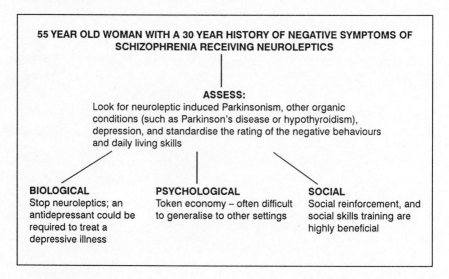

55 YEAR OLD WOMAN WITH A 30 YEAR HISTORY OF NEGATIVE SYMPTOMS OF SCHIZOPHRENIA RECEIVING NEUROLEPTICS

ASSESS:
Look for neuroleptic induced Parkinsonism, other organic conditions (such as Parkinson's disease or hypothyroidism), depression, and standardise the rating of the negative behaviours and daily living skills

BIOLOGICAL
Stop neuroleptics; an antidepressant could be required to treat a depressive illness

PSYCHOLOGICAL
Token economy – often difficult to generalise to other settings

SOCIAL
Social reinforcement, and social skills training are highly beneficial

ASSESSMENT

General opening/special features of the case

There are three parts to the assessment of *chronic schizophrenia*: analysis of the negative symptoms, behaviour, and daily living skills.

Sources of history

The multidisciplinary team.

History and mental state examination

Biological

I would evaluate the severity and consistency of the *negative symp-*

toms, paying particular attention to those of a socially embarrassing nature such as maintaining unusual postures (*catatonia*) or sexual inappropriateness (e.g. public masturbation), and look for any evidence of a *depressive* or *organic condition* which could mimic this negative defect state (such as *neuroleptic-induced Parkinsonism, Parkinson's disease itself, presenile dementia, or hypothyroidism*).

Psychological
A *structured behaviour assessment programme* would be set up by her key nurse and the psychologist – baseline measures of both rewarding activities (such as time off the ward), and undesirable traits (e.g. not cleaning her bed area) would be quantified.

Social
Assessment of her *daily living skills* – especially those related to dressing, personal hygiene, cooking, shopping and motivation could be carried out by the occupational therapist.

Advice about a suitable placement (e.g. half-way house, group house, or hostel) would be requested from the team social (or rehabilitation) officer; it would be essential to discuss the suitability of the placement with her proposed carers before a final decision was made.

Physical examination

I would conduct a thorough physical and neurological examination.

Serological investigations would include a full blood count, liver and thyroid function test, and a syphilis screen.

MANAGEMENT

General opening/special features of the case

The chances of successful rehabilitation would be markedly improved by modification of the negative symptoms of schizophrenia.

Biological
Long-term neuroleptic medication would not only be unlikely to influence the course of her negative symptoms, but would expose her to its chronic side-effects such as *tardive dyskinesia*; I would, therefore, gradually tail off the fluphenazine decanoate. She would require regular review to facilitate the early detection of psychotic symptoms. Any concurrent depressive illness would be helped with a tricyclic antidepressant.

Psychological
Negative behaviours such as poor personal hygiene, could be targeted for modification using a *token economy model*; in practice, however, the gains made using this model could be difficult to sustain in other settings.

Social
Because she has a wide range of negative behaviours including social withdrawal, social skills training, and simple social reinforcement training would be particularly beneficial.

Placement would, primarily, be determined by her optimum level of social readjustment, and the extent to which she could be gradually re-acclimatized to the outside world.

Community care would be carefully planned, and I would be mindful that in a small minority of cases long term institutional care may be the safest and most caring strategy.

REFERENCES AND FURTHER READING

Gelder M, Gath D, Mayou R. *Oxford Textbook of Psychiatry* (second edition). Oxford: Oxford University Press, 1989; chapter 9 p 272–4.

Jones DW, Tomlinson D, Anderson J. Community and asylum care: plus ça change. *Journal of the Royal Society of Medicine* 1991; 252–4.

Rifkin A, Quitkin F, Klein DF. Akinesia. *Archives of General Psychiatry* 1975; 32: 672–4.

Owens DGC, Johnstone EC. The disabilities of chronic schizophrenia. *British Journal of Psychiatry* 1988; 136: 384–95.

Cross reference Question 11A

CHAPTER 12

COMMUNICATING WITH AND HELPING THE CANCER PATIENT

QUESTION 12

You have been asked to see a 40 year old married woman referred by a consultant surgeon because she has been low, anxious, forgetful, waking early, anorexic and losing weight for four months after a mastectomy and radiotherapy for breast cancer. Additionally, she refuses to undress in her husband's presence, and her only close relative has become tired of "trying to cheer her up". The surgeon has assured her that her cancer was detected early and that she has a good prognosis. She, however, does not want to be followed up by her general practitioner whom she describes as a "quack".

What would your management be?

ANSWER 12

See algorithm on next page.

ASSESSMENT

General opening/special features of the case

Management would be dependent on effective communication and assessment of the patient.

Effective communication with the patient would require a willingness to sensitively and genuinely discuss the psychological and physical problems associated with the cancer. Additionally, her relatives would require *education* and *support* to cope with their feelings of *uncertainty* and *helplessness*.

The aim of my assessment would be to determine if her symptoms were an understandable or abnormal psychological reaction to the cancer, or the result of a functional (e.g. depression) or organic (probably due to metastases) mental disorder.

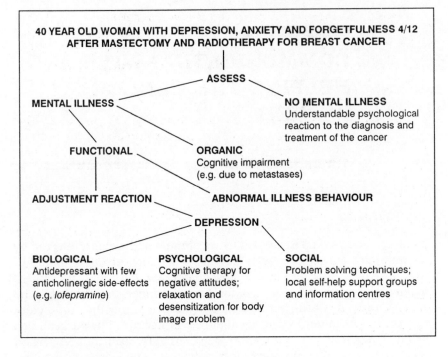

Sources of history

I would arrange to carry out a domiciliary visit accompanied by a member of the *community psychiatric team*.

History and mental state examination

Biological
I would take a history and examine the patient's mental state, and separately, using a *structured family interview*, explore the views of her husband and relatives about her illness.

I would determine the *nature, onset, and progression of her symptoms* and particularly, look for evidence of a *depressive illness* – she has *biological symptoms* (i.e. early morning wakening, appetite and weight loss), and there could be a family history – *ideas of deliberate self harm or suicide*, and *anxiety*.

I would thoroughly investigate the extent of her forgetfulness (anxiety or depression would be more likely precipitants than metastatic disease), and the rest of her cognitive function.[1]

---

1 Cognitive function can be formally tested using the mini-mental state (see Folstein MF, Folstein FE, McHugh PH. "Mini-mental state":. A practical method for grading the cognitive state of patients for the clinician. *Journal of Psychiatric Research* 1975; 12: 189–98.

I would be interested in whether she was receiving any *cytotoxic medication* or *steroids* because of their liability to impair mood, and to exacerbate physical symptoms such as nausea, which could make the patient erroneously conclude that the cancer was spreading.

Psychological

I would, specifically, explore any feelings of:

uncertainty – odd "aches and pains" could be interpreted by the patient and her family as proof of the cancer spreading, therefore if the general practitioner was unable to answer her question satisfactorily or discuss new treatments in detail (an unrealistic expectation) the patient and her family may increase their demands for specialist help;

helplessness – which could lead to passivity;

failure – self-esteem could be impaired by increased reliance on others;

mutilation – which could be responsible for why she can no longer undress in her husband's presence (unsightly scars or a poorly constructed prosthesis could be additional sources of distress, and the *body image problem*[2] could be severe enough to produce psychological neglect of the affected side of the body);

sexual inadequacy – reduction of libido could be a consequence of the body image problem and the loss of self-esteem (often, patients find it difficult to confide in others about such issues and, therefore, sexual difficulty should be directly inquired about);

attribution – the cancer could be falsely regarded as punishment for past failures or personality difficulties, and there could be a *"search for meaning"*.

Social

I would assess the level of support from her friends and relatives, and investigate any suggestion that her symptoms could have been deliberately prolonged or exaggerated (i.e. *abnormal illness behaviour*).

MANAGEMENT

General opening/special features of the case

In general, adjustment disorders are the most common psychological disturbance following mastectomy. In this case, however, the prolonged symptoms with biological features are strongly suggestive of a depressive illness; additionally, radiotherapy following mastectomy and body image problems are known risk factors for depression.

---

2 For an interesting account of body image problems see Sacks O. *The Man Who Mistook his Wife for a Hat*, published by Pan (1986).

Biological
I would select an antidepressant with few anticholinergic[3] side-effects such as *lofepramine* (dose range 70–210 mg daily) to treat the depressive illness, and to provide symptomatic relief of anxiety.

Psychological
I would adopt a *cognitive* approach to deal with her negative self image, and carry out *relaxation* and *desensitization* techniques (to teach her to look at the affected side of her body). The need for *marital or sex therapy* would be carefully considered.

Social
Problem-solving techniques could be directed at issues of concern in the family identified by the structured interview. Attendance at a local support[4] group or leisure club would be encouraged.

REFERENCES AND FURTHER READING

Gautam S, Nijhawan M. Communicating with cancer patients. *British Journal of Psychiatry* 1987; 150: 760–4.

Gelder M, Gath D, Mayou R. *Oxford Textbook of Psychiatry* (second edition). Oxford: Oxford University Press, 1989; chapter 12 p 462–4.

MacGuire P. The psychological impact of cancer. *British Journal of Hospital Medicine* (August) 1985: 100–3.

---

3 The profound anticholinergic side-effects of first generation tricyclic antidepressants such as amitriptyline or imipramine can mimic the presenting symptoms of cancer.
4 Information about local support groups can be obtained from the Breast Care and Mastectomy Association of Great Britain 28A Kings Cross London WC1 8JG (Telephone: 071–837–0908).

CHAPTER 13

BEREAVEMENT AND THE PSYCHOLOGICAL CARE OF THE DYING

QUESTION 13A

You have been asked to see a 30 year old widow whose husband died suddenly of a myocardial infarction nine months ago, shortly after they had been quarrelling. Their relationship had always been a difficult one, and shortly before his death she had been planning to start divorce proceedings, but had not told him. She did not feel sad when he died, and did not attend his funeral. For the last three months (six months after her husband's death), she has, however, been complaining of crying a lot; feeling depressed; waking early in the morning; anxious; off her food; and has not been able to get him out of her mind or come to terms with his death.

How would you manage this problem?

ANSWER 13A

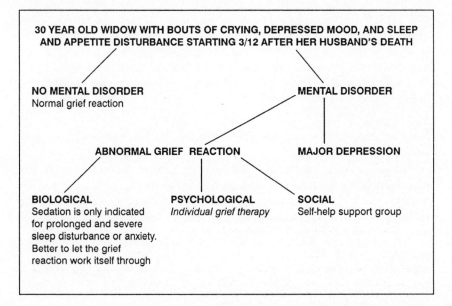

30 YEAR OLD WIDOW WITH BOUTS OF CRYING, DEPRESSED MOOD, AND SLEEP AND APPETITE DISTURBANCE STARTING 3/12 AFTER HER HUSBAND'S DEATH

NO MENTAL DISORDER
Normal grief reaction

MENTAL DISORDER

ABNORMAL GRIEF REACTION

MAJOR DEPRESSION

BIOLOGICAL
Sedation is only indicated for prolonged and severe sleep disturbance or anxiety. Better to let the grief reaction work itself through

PSYCHOLOGICAL
Individual grief therapy

SOCIAL
Self-help support group

ASSESSMENT

General opening/special features of the case

Management is dependent on assessment.

The factors which, taken together, point to an *abnormal* (*complicated and delayed*) *grief reaction*, in contrast to a *normal grief reaction*, are: the suddenness of her husband's death; her strong feelings of anger towards him; her refusal to attend his funeral or to properly say "goodbye"; and the delayed onset of her symptoms. I would, however, have to exclude a *major depressive illness*.

Sources of history

I would interview the patient, and separately, a close friend or relative.

History and mental state examination

I would look for a family or personal history of depression; such people frequently respond to a loss or bereavement with a major depressive illness.

Biological symptoms, such as early morning wakening and appetite loss are common to both a major depression and a grief reaction. I would therefore, in addition, search for symptoms which would discriminate between them. These include: *marked guilt*; persistent *delusions* or *hallucinations of being evil or wicked*, or of having caused her husband's death; *severe functional impairment*; and *ideas of worthlessness or suicide* are suggestive of a major depression. In contrast, the grieving process is usually associated with: *emotionality*, *changes of mood* from sadness to increasing pleasure from activities as time goes by; a search for, and a response to sympathetic gestures; *self-blame* (restricted to specific acts of commission or omission); and *dreams, persistent thoughts*, or *fleeting illusions or hallucinations of being in the deceased's presence*.

Psychological
I would explore the *defence mechanisms* she has employed to *deny* her *anger* and *loss*.

Has she: been uncharacteristically euphoric; taken on any of the characteristics or mannerisms of her husband (*identification phenomena*), as if to perpetuate his existence; or has she *displaced* her feelings to some other situation, like immersing herself in, or overreacting to someone else's troubles?

Social
I would ascertain whether she had been *isolated* or *neglected* by her friends or had *withdrawn* herself from social activities; she may, therefore, be feeling lonely, unsupported, or rejected.

MANAGEMENT

General opening/special features of the case

The most likely diagnosis is of an *abnormal grief reaction*.

Biological
Unless there is prolonged and severe sleep disturbance or anxiety, I would not interfere with the grieving process by prescribing sedative drugs; antidepressants or antianxiety agents would only be dispensed if there was a concurrent major depressive illness or anxiety state.

Psychological
To set up a *therapeutic alliance* in *grief therapy*, it would be essential for me to convey to her that I was comfortable about dealing with issues about death and dying, and capable of coping with the strong feelings of anger and self-blame which would occur as she started to talk openly about her husband, handle items of his clothing, or visit his grave. During the preliminary sessions, I would, perhaps, at first have to be an active therapist, but as her confidence and self-esteem improved, I would encourage her to take up her responsibilities and plan for the future.

Social
I would advise her to accept emotional support from close friends or family if it is offered. This, however, may not be practicable, given that there may be some family tensions, or hostility towards her for not attending her husband's funeral which may not be easily resolved. Thus, I would suggest that she join a local self-help group[1] which would offer friendship, new social contacts, and a way of re-introducing herself back into society.

REFERENCES AND FURTHER READING

Freud S. Mourning and melancholia (1917). In the *Standard Edition of the Complete Works of Sigmund Freud*. London: Hogarth Press, 1957 Volume 14.

Gelder M, Gath D, Mayou R. *Oxford Textbook of Psychiatry* (second edition). Oxford: Oxford University Press, 1989: chapter 8 p 226–7.

Kutscher A, Carr A, Kutscher L. *Principles of Thanatology*. New York: Columbia University Press, 1987.

Parkes CM. Bereavement, *British Journal of Psychiatry*, 1985; 146: 11–7.

---

1 An example of a self-help group is one run by CRUSE.

QUESTION 13B

You have been asked to see a 45 year old married man at a local hospice who was diagnosed as having carcinoma of the lung a month ago. His doctors felt it was kind not to give him too many details about his illness because it might upset him, and in any case, he had not himself raised any questions about it. Physically, he is often breathless and nauseous, but not in pain. Recently, his behaviour has changed: He has been shouting at the nurses at the hospice who report that he is sleeping poorly, depressed and anxious. Frequently, he says he wants to go home and has never felt better, but becomes distressed when his wife and children visit him.

How would you manage this problem?

ANSWER 13B

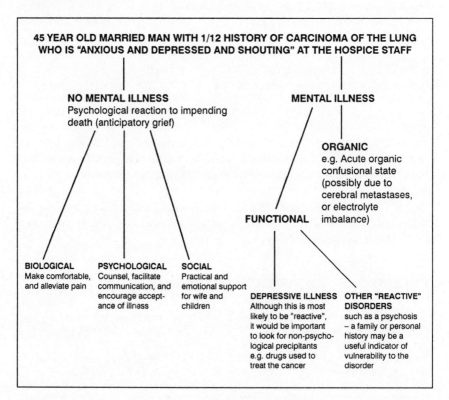

ASSESSMENT

General opening/special features of the case

Management is dependent on assessment.

This relatively young man with dependents is having to face an untimely death which he probably expects to be unpleasant, painful or undignified. He has not received sufficient information about his prognosis, nor has he been given the opportunity to put his affairs in order.

My assessment would determine whether his behaviour and symptoms were an understandable psychological reaction to the anticipated loss of friends, family, and of his own future (*anticipatory grief*), or the result of a functional (usually depressive) or organic mental illness.

Sources of history

I would interview the patient and his wife, separately at first, and then together, and his key worker at the hospice.

History and mental state examination

Biological
I would be interested in a past family or personal history of mental illness (especially of depression).

I would explore the onset and progression of his symptoms. I would specifically look for: *biological symptoms of depression*; symptoms of *anxiety* or *panic* (with which the dyspnoea could be associated); evidence of any other mental disorder which could have been triggered by the acute stress of his illness such as a reactive psychosis; and test his cognitive function – *acute organic confusional states* due to electrolyte imbalance or cerebral metastases are common.

Psychological
I would ascertain, from his premorbid personality, how he coped and reacted to stress in the past, and what his outlook on life was.

I would determine, by allowing him to lead the discussion, how much he knew or wished to know about his illness, and whether he could come to terms with his *defence mechanisms of denial*, and *displacement of guilt and anger* towards the hospice workers.

Social
I would assess the level of family support, and, sensitively, inquire about whether he had made a will, or had any last wishes.

MANAGEMENT

General opening/special features of the case

The diagnosis is of *anticipatory grief*.

I would help him to calmly accept the reality of his illness and its prognosis, and attend to his comfort. "The person should be relatively free from pain, should operate on as effective a level as possible, should recognise and resolve remaining conflicts, should satisfy as far as possible remaining wishes and should be able to yield control to others in whom he has confidence" (Hackett and Weissman, 1962).

Biological
I would make him as comfortable as I could by paying particular attention to adequate pain relief, and reviewing the necessity of any drugs which could have an adverse effect on his mental state.

Psychological
I would try to develop a trusting relationship with him which would allow us to have open and frank discussions about his illness and his projected feelings of anger towards the staff. To gain his confidence, I would be non-judgemental and tolerant. And I would help him to *communicate* more effectively with both the staff and his family, who could themselves be uncertain or may simply not know how to talk to someone who was dying.

I would encourage him to: actively participate in decisions about his care; try and accept his illness and to yield some control to the staff (*partial dependency*); properly say "*goodbye*".

Social
I would offer what support I could to the hospice staff.

A social worker would be needed to provide socio-economic advice – important issues to cover would include making a will, fulfilling last wishes if possible, discussing how the family would cope with his death and the resolution of any outstanding interpersonal or intra-familial conflicts.

REFERENCES AND FURTHER READING

Gelder M, Gath D, Mayou R. *Oxford Textbook of Psychiatry* (second edition). Oxford: Oxford University Press, 1989; chapter 12 p 426–9.

Hackett TP, Weissman A. The treatment of the dying. *Current Psychiatric Therapy* 1962; 2: 121–6.

Kubler-Ross E. *On Death and Dying*. New York: Macmillan, 1969.

Leming MR, Dickinson GE. *Understanding Dying, Death and Bereavement*. New York: Holt, Rinehart and Winston, 1985.

Parkes CM. Care of the dying: the role of the psychiatrist. *British Journal of Hospital Medicine* (October) 1986: 250–5.

QUESTION 13C

You are on a liaison psychiatry attachment covering the accident and emergency department. While in the department, a ten year old girl is brought in with severe injuries from which she later dies. The parents, who were also in the car, but were unhurt, have been in the patients' waiting area all along.

How would you "break the news"?

How would you deal with this situation?

ANSWER 13C

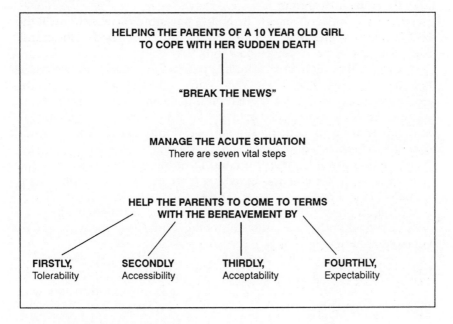

"BREAKING THE NEWS"

General opening

The sudden death of a child is usually a devastating emotional experience for the parents. I would expect that the child's parents would, at first, *react with shock, disbelief, confusion or anger*, and could also feel resentful towards me as the bearer of bad news; additionally, they could be feeling *guilty because they survived*. Furthermore, there is the disadvantage that a professional relationship has not had time to form.

"Breaking the news" has two parts: the management of the immediate situation in the department, and helping the child's parents to come to terms with the bereavement.

Management of the acute situation

Before "breaking the news", I would move the child's parents to a *private room* where we would not be disturbed. Because I would have to support them through this without becoming defensive myself, it would be helpful if I could *share this responsibility* with a colleague in authority (e.g. a chaplain, doctor, nurse, or social worker).

Firstly, my colleague and I would aim to reduce the trauma of the death by assuring the parents that the child did not suffer unnecessarily; was not left alone; and that all that could be done, was done. It would be most appropriate to deliver this in a sympathetic and informative manner.

Next, we would encourage the child's parents to see the body; if the body is badly mutilated, the parents would be warned beforehand, and given the opportunity to postpone this.

Thirdly, we would offer the child's parents the chance of preparing the child for burial.

Fourthly, we would place great emphasis on allowing the parents as much time as they needed to overcome this "numbness" and shock, and rather than pressuring speech, we would *concentrate on small acts of kindness* such as providing nourishment.

Fifthly, we would invite the parents to tell us about the last few hours of the child's life, and to ask us more detailed questions about how the child died.

Sixthly, we would arrange to meet with other members of staff who were involved with caring for the child, and allow them to openly ventilate their feelings.

Seventhly, we would, sympathetically, decline any request for tranquillisers or sleeping tablets; instead, we would offer to be available to support them, and to help them to come to terms with their bereavement.

Coming to terms with bereavement

There are four principles to managing sudden death. They are: *tolerability* – reducing the impact; *accessibility* – significant others are allowed to provide practical and emotional support; *acceptability* – realising that everyone will die, gradually letting go, resolving problems, and returning to reality; and *expectability* – realising that nobody's time of death is predictable.

Thus, we would plan to see the child's parents, preferably the following day, to: find out where they were in terms of their feelings; *educate them about the "normality" of their grief*, and to know what to expect and get by without developing unhealthy *coping mechanisms*; and to discuss *practical arrangements* such as arranging the funeral.

At a pre-arranged time in the future, usually between three and six months, we would meet to explore any "forgotten" issues or new developments (it would be important to look for any evidence of an *unresolved grief reaction*, or a *depressive illness*); alternatively, the parents might prefer to do this work with their general practitioner, priest or some other counsellor with whom they have an established relationship.

REFERENCES AND FURTHER READING

Cassem NH. Treating the person confronting death. In: *The Harvard Guide to Modern Psychiatry*, Nicholi Jr AM (editor). Cambridge: Harvard University Press, 1978.

Weisman AD. Coping with untimely death. *Psychiatry* 1973; 36: 366–78.

CHAPTER 14

SEXUAL PROBLEMS AND SEXUAL IDENTITY

QUESTION 14A

You have been asked by a consultant surgeon to see a twenty year old man who wishes to change his sex. He tells you he has always known he was the wrong sex and feels his external genitalia are repugnant. He has also been dressing in female clothes since the age of eight. How would you assess him in order to reach a differential diagnosis?

What would your management be if he requested a sex change operation?

ANSWER 14A

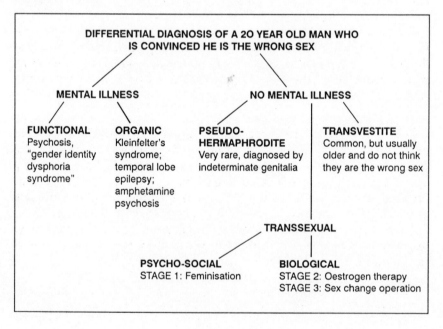

ASSESSMENT

General opening/special features of the case

Because the patient may have invested a lot of hope in the first meeting, or may be expecting an immediate decision, I would warn him that the assessment would be detailed, perhaps prolonged, and certainly on-going.

Sources of history

I would wish to interview the patient himself, and reliable informants, especially those who have known him from birth. Pictures and photographic tapes (if available) of the patient's early life and development would be useful.

History and mental state examination

Biological
I would look for any evidence in his obstetric or developmental history of: prenatal or perinatal illnesses or operations; exposure to feminising hormones; and ascertain his birth weight and developmental milestones.

I would observe his mannerisms related to gender role; and look for a: past family or personal history of mental illness; current mental illness – especially of *psychosis* or *antisocial personality disorder* – which could be responsible[1] for the cross-dressing behaviour; or a *"reactive" depression* or *anxiety state*.

Psychological
I would ascertain: the exact age at which the patient started to cross-dress; the first time he wished for a change of sex; and the details of his sexual development – for example, did he have any spontaneous erections or emissions? What was his level of sexual arousal[2] while cross-dressing? What were his masturbatory fantasies or fetishes? Did he have any sadistic or homosexual tendencies?

I would formally assess his personality. Baseline psychometric tests of intelligence and attitude[3] would also be essential; serial ratings would provide objective indicators of change.

---

1 *Gender identity dysphoria syndrome* is an emotional state of anxiety, depression, and restlessness" which occurs in people who are chronically unhappy about their sexual role and thus, request a sex change. Up to six subtypes have been described (see Hampson JL 1974).

2 Transvestites, unlike transsexuals, are sexually aroused by cross-dressing.

3 Examples of standard psychometric tests for intelligence, personality and attitude include the *Weschler Adult Intelligence Scale,* the *Eysenck Personality Questionnaire* and the *Terman-Miles Attitude-interest Test.*

Social

I would examine the attitude of his parents to his: conception and birth (e.g. were they pleased, or was it an unfortunate "accident"); current gender identity (i.e. was this encouraged or discouraged?); and assess the quality of their *parenting style* – was there any evidence of excessive passivity or dominance by either parent?

And I would determine his level of *social adjustment* – what explanation did he give for his sexual orientation and cross dressing? How did he relate to members of his own sex or of the opposite sex? What social consequences has expressing his sexuality brought about (e.g. losing his job or friends)?

Physical examination

I would examine his external genitalia, look for secondary sexual characteristics, and arrange a skull and chest X-ray, genetic screen, and electroencephalogram. Other investigations would include measurements of serum follicle stimulating hormone (FSH), luteinizing hormone (LH), and testosterone.

Differential diagnosis
See algorithm.

MANAGEMENT

General opening/special features of the case

Before implementing a management plan to change his sexual identity, I would ensure that he: was aware it was a life long commitment; had not underestimated the amount of social readjustment he would have to face; or overestimated the benefit of a sex change operation to his quality of life.

Supportive psychotherapy would be offered regardless of whether or not the request for a sex change was granted.

There would be three steps to changing his sexual identity.

Psycho-social
STAGE 1: I would arrange for him to learn, using *behaviour modification techniques*, appropriate feminine gestures, speech delivery, dress style, and fine details of comportment – for example, how to apply make up, remove facial hair (electrolysis would be recommended), adopt appropriate body postures, walk, and socially interact with men.

Guidance on how to seek appropriate professional help with practical issues such as changing his name, or obtaining a new driving licence or passport would be given; marriage to another man is currently not legally permissible in the United Kingdom.

Biological

STAGE 2: Before starting oestrogen[4] treatment (stilboestrol 0.25–0.5 mg/day to give him a more feminine appearance, I would warn him of its health risks.

STAGE 3: If he was able to live as a woman for at least a year, and his personality has remained stable, I would give permission for the sex change operation to proceed.

REFERENCES AND FURTHER READING

Gelder M, Gath D, Mayou R. *Oxford Textbook of Psychiatry* (second edition) Oxford: Oxford University Press 1989; Chapter 15 p 590–95.

Green R, Money J. *Transsexualism and Sex Reassignment*. Baltimore: John Hopkins Press, 1969.

Hampson JL. In: *Proceedings of the Interdisciplinary Symposium on Gender Dysphoria Syndrome*, Grandy P and Lamb D (editors), Ann Arbor: Edwards Brothers, 1974.

Morris J. *Conundrum*. London: Faber and Faber, 1974.

Snaith P. Gender reassignment today. *British Medical Journal* 1987; 295:454.

Walinder J. Transsexualism – definition, prevalence and sex distribution. *Acta Psychiatrica et Neurologica Scandinavica* 1968; supplement 203: 255–8.

---

4 Some patients on oestrogen therapy report weepiness and lability of mood – interestingly, this makes some patients feel more feminine. Dangerous side-effects of oestrogen therapy include thrombosis and an increased risk of breast cancer.

QUESTION 14B

A 36 year old married civil servant, with no apparent premorbid personality maladjustment or past psychiatric history, has become panic-stricken shortly after being coerced to visit a male brothel, for the first time, with a friend. He is convinced that everyone now knows he is gay. As evidence, he cites that while attending a conference the following week, a male colleague with whom he was sharing a room was intentionally bumping in to him.

Could you very briefly list the possibilities?

ANSWER 14B

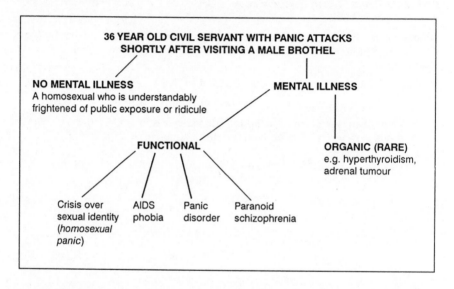

DIFFERENTIAL DIAGNOSIS

His symptoms could be related to, or independent of mental illness.

If there was *no mental illness*, he could be a homosexual with an understandable fear of public exposure or ridicule by his friend.

If there was evidence of a *mental illness*, the cause could be either functional (neurotic or psychotic) or organic.

The likely neurotic disorders would include: a state of severe anxiety precipitated by confusion over his *sexual identity*, often loosely, and controversially, termed as *homosexual panic* (i.e. the civil servant was, basically, heterosexual, but had repressed homosexual drives, the resistance to which may have been lowered by alcohol or drugs); *AIDS phobia* (i.e. anxiety and rumination about having contracted the human immunodeficiency virus); and a *de nouveau* but coincidental *panic disorder* with generalised anxiety.

The important psychotic disorders to exclude would be a *brief reactive psychosis* to the trauma of the experience, and a *paranoid psychosis*, such as paranoid schizophrenia which could have either predated the visit to the brothel or been triggered by it and to which he could be vulnerable by virtue of a past family or personal history.

An organic cause would be rare in a man of this age, and related to those disorders which could provoke anxiety; thus, it would be essential to exclude *hyperthyroidism* or an *adrenal tumour*.

REFERENCES AND FURTHER READING

Chaung HT, Addington D. Homosexual panic: A review of its concept. *Canadian Journal of Psychiatry* 1988; 33: 613-7.

Gonsiorek JC. *The Use of Diagnostic Concepts in Working with Gay and Lesbian Populations: Homosexuality and Psychotherapy – A Practitioner's Handbook of Affirmative Models* 1982(7): 2 and 3.

Ovesey L. *Homosexuality and Pseudohomosexuality*. New York: Science, 1969.

QUESTION 14C

You have been asked by a general practitioner to assess a 55 year old businessman whose wife has urged him to seek help for erectile impotence.

How would you proceed?

What is the most likely outcome?

What would your management be?

ANSWER14C

See algorithm on next page

ASSESSMENT

General opening/special features of the case

My aims would be to: determine whether the problem was *physical*, *psychological*, or *both* and to chart its development; *educate* the couple; establish a *therapeutic relationship*; and to assess their suitability for treatment.

A sensitive but frank approach would be required to get the couple to relax. And it is often worthwhile to let them know the length of the session at the start of the initial interview to reduce any anxieties of having to rush; additionally, the assessment may have to take place over several sessions.

I would, and if possible with a co-therapist[5], interview the patient and his wife separately, and then together to find out how they relate to each other and to formulate a treatment plan. We would allocate ourselves the same-sex partner, and assure them of confidentiality about what they do not wish to be disclosed to the other partner.

History and mental state examination

Physical

I would be interested in the *onset, nature and progression of the symptoms*. And in particular, whether an erection: was possible in any situation (he could be potent with a mistress but not his wife); when it occurred was partial, total, misshapen (as in Peyronie's disease), or associated with a particular part of sexual activity (e.g. penetration); was achievable and sustainable on his own by fantasies or masturbation; ever happened in his sleep, or on waking up in the morning (which would suggest the impotence was psychological rather than physical in origin).

---

5 Co-therapists are not wholly essential, but experience suggests that they can provide useful alternative insights, particularly with treatment-resistant cases.

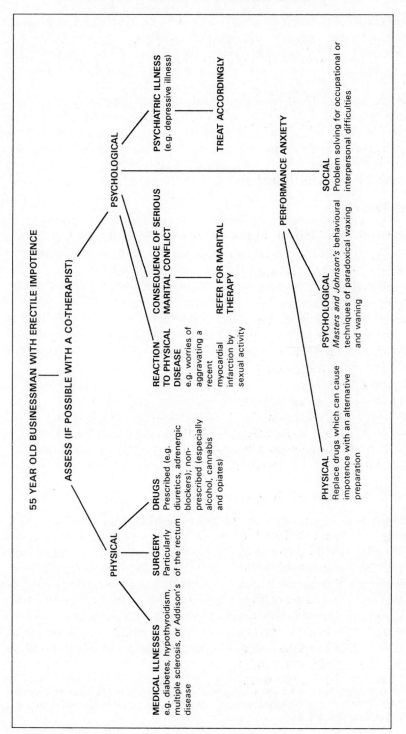

Because the erectile impotence could be related to a *physical disorder* in the man, I would specifically inquire about any: medical illnesses, such as nervous system damage by diabetes mellitus or multiple sclerosis, peripheral vascular damage by arteriosclerosis, or endocrine disorder as in Addison's disease. Other causes of impotence include: anxiety that sexual intercourse would aggravate a physical illness such as a recent myocardial infarction; surgical operations which damage the nerve supply to the perineum or peri-anal area; prescribed drugs (e.g. thiazide diuretics, or adrenergic blockers); and non-prescribed drugs especially alcohol, cannabis, or opiates – thus, a carefully taken drug and alcohol history would be essential.

Psychological
In both partners, it would be important to look for: *predisposing factors* in early life to sexual difficulties (e.g a strict upbringing, intrafamilial conflict, or insufficient sexual information, insecurity about sexual roles or identity); *precipitants* (e.g. infidelity, other interpersonal difficulties[6], or a psychiatric disorder such as depression); and *perpetuating factors* (e.g. performance anxiety, serious marital problems, loss of sexual interest, guilt, or a fear of intimacy).

And the primary sexual difficulty could be his wife's (e.g. vaginismus); thus, his impotence could be due to anticipatory anxiety about hurting his wife.

Social
In the man, I would look for evidence of social pressures such as financial difficulty, overwork, or stressful life events which could impair his performance; similar pressures on his wife could result in a loss of sexual interest or enthusiasm which could inhibit his arousal.

Physical examination

The physical examination of the man would be thorough and methodical.

I would: *firstly*, look for general signs of a physical illness, with particular emphasis on excluding diabetes, hypertension, and arteriosclerosis (funduscopic and neurological examination would be essential), and thyroid disease. Increased skin pigmentation, hair loss or gynaecomastia could be indicators of Addison's disease.

Secondly, examine the external genitalia (penis and testicles) for abnormalities in shape, size or sensitivity, and for signs of disease

---

6 Interpersonal difficulties could be uncovered by exploring the quality of the relationship. This includes assessment of the commitment, communication, contextual threat of a stressful event such as an argument, conflict resolution, and caring (the 5 C's).

such as plaques (as in *Peyronie's disease*) or a urethral discharge due to infection;

thirdly, perform a serological screen – thyroid and liver function tests, fasting glucose, testosterone (and prolactin if the testosterone is low), luteinizing hormone, and adrenocorticotrophic hormone;

fourthly, carefully consider the need for specialised examinations to confirm penile rigidity – for instance, a *nocturnal penile tumescence strain gauge*.

Outcome
Erectile impotence is most likely to have been psychologically induced by performance anxiety after a period of normal function.

MANAGEMENT

General opening/special features of the case

Assuming there were no severe interpersonal conflicts for which marital therapy would be more appropriate, and the couple were motivated, I would adopt the treatment technique pioneered by *Masters and Johnson*. This technique has four characteristic features: treating the couple together, improving their communication, educating them about the anatomy and physiology of sexual intercourse, and setting graded sexual tasks (homework).

Physical
Drugs which could cause impotence should be replaced by an alternative preparation and any concurrent physical illness should be treated.

Specific treatments[7] such as the production of "chemical" erections would not be indicated where the cause was psychological.

Psychological
A fixed number of treatment sessions would be allocated. The woman would be directed, in a graded fashion, to progress from non-genital to genital sensate focusing during which time her husband would, paradoxically, be told (i.e. *paradoxical intention*) not to have an erection to take the pressure off him. Intercourse would be banned. The couple would be advised to use a lotion while caressing, and the man would be asked to concentrate on receiving pleasure.

If this procedure was unsuccessful, erotic fantasies, and if acceptable, oral stimulation would be encouraged. Once the programme sensate focusing starts to produce strong erections[8], the woman

---

7 Specific treatments, such as the injection of alpha-bungarotoxin into the penis to produce a "chemical" erection or the implantation of a prosthesis, have been used where the erectile dysfunction was due to physical causes.

8 Erections are more readily achievable early in the morning or on waking.

should stop caressing and wait for the erection to subside before restarting. The *waxing and waning* technique would be used to build the man's confidence.

When penetration becomes permissible, the woman should take charge and insert his penis, to reduce any anxiety associated with penetration.

Social
The use of *problem-solving techniques* to address social pressures (e.g. overwork), lifestyle, or minor interpersonal problems would be encouraged.

REFERENCES AND FURTHER READING

Gelder M, Gath D, Mayou R. *Oxford Textbook of Psychiatry* (second edition). Oxford: Oxford University Press, 1989; chapter 15 p 565 and 570–3.

Hawton K. *Sex Therapy: a Practical Guide*. Oxford: Oxford University Press, 1985.

Masters WH, Johnson VE. *Human Sexual Inadequacy*. London: Churchill, 1970.

CHAPTER 15

OBSESSIVE–COMPULSIVE DISORDER

QUESTION 15A

A 24 year old female nurse is referred to you for repeatedly washing her hands because of a constant worry that they are dirty. A month ago, she had the unfortunate experience of looking after a patient who died of meningitis. She has also been tearful, but eating and sleeping normally.

How would you assess her, and what are the possible explanations of her symptoms? What would your management be?

ANSWER 15A

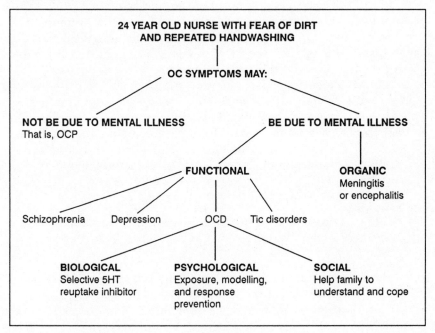

24 YEAR OLD NURSE WITH FEAR OF DIRT
AND REPEATED HANDWASHING

OC SYMPTOMS MAY:

NOT BE DUE TO MENTAL ILLNESS
That is, OCP

BE DUE TO MENTAL ILLNESS

FUNCTIONAL

ORGANIC
Meningitis
or encephalitis

Schizophrenia   Depression   OCD   Tic disorders

BIOLOGICAL
Selective 5HT
reuptake inhibitor

PSYCHOLOGICAL
Exposure, modelling,
and response
prevention

SOCIAL
Help family to
understand and cope

ASSESSMENT

General opening/special features of the case

The aim of my assessment would be to determine whether the obsessive–compulsive (OC) symptoms were either *egosyntonic*, that is, due to an obsessive-compulsive personality (OCP) or *egodystonic*, the result of a mental disorder such as obsessive–compulsive disorder (OCD) or *depression*.

Sources of history

I would interview the patient and separately, a close member of the family.

History and mental state examination

Biological
I would look for a family or personal history of mental illness, particularly of *OCD* or *depression*.

I would find out: the frequency of the handwashing; whether the thoughts to wash her hands were *resisted* and the accompanying *emotional tone* (e.g. anxiety); and examine the progression of her symptoms – that is, have the OC symptoms been persistently troublesome, or have they fluctuated in intensity?

I would, specifically, look for current evidence of a depressive illness (with *biological symptoms*), which may have worsened or given rise to the OC symptoms, and exclude other psychiatric disorders with which the OC symptoms may, although less frequently, be linked. Functional disorders would include *schizophrenia* and *tic disorders* (including *Tourette syndrome*); organic causes would include *meningitis* or *encephalitis*.

Psychological
I would be interested in her interpretation of the symptoms, and the *defence mechanisms*[1] she has used to cope with them.

Social
I would ascertain the impact of the symptoms on her life style (e.g. Has she been able to return to work? Have the symptoms brought about any interpersonal or sexual difficulties? How have the family coped, and do they understand the nature of her symptoms? Have the family resisted or colluded with her symptoms in any way?).

---

1 The defence mechanisms commonly associated with OCD include magical undoing, isolation, and reaction formation.

Explanation of symptoms

See algorithm.

MANAGEMENT

General opening/special features of the case

The most likely diagnosis is of OCD and depression.

Frequently, it is necessary to assure the patient that her OC symptoms are not "a sign of madness". I would start treatment on an outpatient basis, but if the symptoms prove to be intractable; a short period of in-patient treatment would be undertaken.

The advice of a behavioural psychologist would also be required.

Biological

I would start her on a selective 5HT reuptake inhibitor such as *fluoxetine* or *fluvoxamine*.

Psychological

With the advice of a behavioural psychologist, I would commence a *graded behaviour programme*. She would: *be exposed* to dirt; get to handle the dirt by *modelling* herself on my doing it and, at the same time, she would be prevented from escaping from the situation and from *handwashing* (i.e. *response prevention*).

Social

For the behavioural programme to be successful, her family would have to: be educated about her symptoms; reinforce the behavioural programme and not collude with her breaking the rules; provide emotional support and encouragement.

REFERENCES AND FURTHER READING

Beech HR. *Obsessional States*. London: Methuen, 1974.

Gelder M, Gath D, Mayou R. *Oxford Textbook of Psychiatry* (second edition). Oxford : Oxford University Press, 1989 chapter 7 p 196–202.

Montgomery SA, Goodman WK, Geoting N. *Obsessive-Compulsive Disorder*. Hampshire: Duphar Medical Relations, 1990.

Rachman S, Hodgson RJ. *Obsessions and Compulsions*. New Jersey: Prentice-Hall, 1980.

QUESTION 15B

You have been asked to see a 40 year old housewife who has suffered from severe obsessions for the last 10 years. She has had intensive pharmacotherapy and behavioural treatment without success.

What other treatment is there? How would you discuss its relative merits, and if she agrees to treatment, what criteria would she have to fulfil?

ANSWER 15B

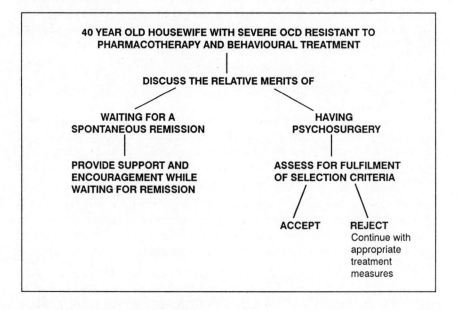

ALTERNATIVE TREATMENTS

The possibilities are *psychosurgery*, or waiting for a *spontaneous remission*.

"BREAKING THE NEWS"

Psychosurgery still, unfortunately, carries in most people's minds, the connotation of being made docile or rendered "a vegetable".

The topic would, therefore, be brought up not only with great tact, but with openness. And I would be prepared to spend time (over several sessions) *educating* her, and responding to her concerns. Because she could be surprised or anxious at the meeting, I would advise that she brought her husband along for support, and to help with the recall of important details. It would be fair to warn her that the procedure for obtaining permission to carry out the operation, should she be willing, could be lengthy. Additionally, she would have to submit to an examination by the neurosurgeon who would undertake the operation; I would advise her to meet him, to discuss the procedure, before making her decision.

I would tell her about the relative merits of the operation in relation to her illness: obsessive-compulsive disorder (OCD) follows a fluctuating course with remissions; there is, therefore, the possibility, but no guarantee, that she could get better without any treatment. However, because of the low 'placebo' response to treatment of OCD, specific treatments such as psychosurgery could be more beneficial than less specific supportive measures.

There are no controlled studies (prevented by ethical considerations) of the efficacy of psychosurgery in OCD. The results of open studies are, however, encouraging (78% of patients show some improvement), but because they are largely based on clinical impressions, may be subject to bias. Improvement is often gradual, and could take up to two years. During this time, intensive behavioural and interpersonal psychotherapy would have to continue.

With modern neurosurgical techniques, *stereotactic surgery*, the risk of side-effects such as increased wakefulness, sensitivity to drugs or alcohol, intracerebral haemorrhage, epilepsy, and personality change, is small.

The decision about whether or not to go ahead would, of course, be hers, and she should take all the time she needs to discuss it with relatives and friends before coming to a decision.

SELECTION CRITERIA

Firstly, she fulfils the first criterion of having incapacitating symptoms for more than five years, and also the *second* and *third*: that pharmacological and behavioural treatments respectively, had failed to alleviate her OCD.

Fourthly, I would ensure that there were no unresolved personal or family conflicts maintaining the illness.

Fifthly, she should not be dependent on drugs or alcohol (as tolerance to these would be reduced by the operation).

Sixthly, she should have no history of antisocial or aggressive behaviour.

Seventhly, she should have no co-existing organic brain disease.

And *eighthly*, because it is a treatment requiring consent and a second opinion, under section 57 of the 1983 Mental Health Act, she would need to submit her case to a *Mental Health Review Tribunal* (comprised of a psychiatrist, a lay person, and a lawyer) for permission.

REFERENCES AND FURTHER READING

Bartlett J, Bridges P, Kelly D. Contemporary indications for psychosurgery. *British Journal of Psychiatry* 1981; 138: 507–11.

Claire AJ. Psychosurgery. In: *Psychiatry in Dissent*, p 278–342. London: Tavistock.

Cobb J, Kelly D. Psychosurgery: is it ever justified? In: *Dilemmas and Difficulties in the Management of Psychiatric Patients*. Hawton K, Cowen P (editors). Oxford: Oxford University Press, 1990.

Gelder M, Gath D, Mayou R. *Oxford Textbook of Psychiatry* (second edition). Oxford: Oxford University Press, 1989; chapter 17 p 689–9

CHAPTER 16

PSYCHOLOGICAL MANAGEMENT OF MEDICAL AND SURGICAL PATIENTS

QUESTION 16A

You have been asked by a consultant plastic surgeon to see a young woman of 22 who has been demanding cosmetic surgery on her nose which she believes to be deformed.
   (a) How would you manage the problem?
   (b) Will you advise the surgeon to carry out the surgery?

ANSWER 16A

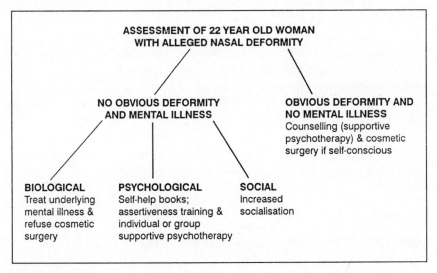

ASSESSMENT

General opening/special features of the case

Whether or not the patient has an obvious nasal deformity, she could have some reservations at seeing a psychiatrist for what she could perceive as, essentially, a "physical problem". And such patients have usually been "passed on" by several specialists. Thus, I would be mindful that she could be ambivalent, suspicious, or even resentful towards doctors – a supportive, sympathetic interview style, giving assurances where possible, would be essential.

Sources of history

Prior to my interview with the patient, I would speak to the plastic surgeon to: obtain more clinical details (particularly about the surgical chances of success); determine his/her expectations of what my interview with the patient was likely to achieve and establish how the decision to ask for a psychiatric opinion was arrived at (including her attitudes about it). I would also be keen to interview the patient's partner, if she has one and consents to this, separately at first, and afterwards, in her company.

History and mental state examination

Biological

I would take a history and examine her mental state. Specifically, I would look for evidence of a *depressive illness, monosymptomatic delusion, schizophrenia* or a *paranoid psychosis*. It would be important to exclude *obsessive-compulsive disorder*.

Psychological

I would be interested in: her opinion of the impact of her nasal deformity on her life; whether her expectations of surgery were realistic – for example, she could erroneously believe that the operation would markedly improve her appearance, or magically solve the difficulties in a personal relationship (especially a sexual problem); any evidence of an abnormal personality or low self-esteem.

Social

I would like to know if her beliefs concerning her nose have increased her anxiety in social settings; a consequence of which may be social withdrawal.

MANAGEMENT

General opening/special features of the case

At the end of the assessment, I would come to a conclusion about whether the beliefs about her nose were clearly excessive (false); and whether there was any other evidence of mental illness.

If there is an obvious nasal deformity and no evidence of mental illness such as a depressive illness, counselling (supportive psychotherapy) should be offered; a *Rogerian* approach, dealing with "here and now", could be a useful technique. If the deformity would be improved by surgery, and she feels self-conscious about it, permission should be given for this to proceed.

If there is minimal or no obvious abnormality (i.e. dysmorpho-phobia), I would tactfully decline her request for surgery and offer to help with the mental abnormality.

Biological
I would treat any mental illness in the appropriate way.

Psychological
The difficulties are often compounded by low self-esteem and inter-personal problems. These need help. Counselling and providing self-help books[1] may be all that is needed. For more entrenched difficul-ties, I would include *assertiveness training* sessions and encourage attendance at a support group. More specific help may be needed with inter-personal, sexual or occupational problems.

Social
If she has withdrawn from social contacts, I would give practical advice such as joining local or activity clubs; she may need to be chaperoned, preferably by her partner or a friend, or exposed in a graded fashion to these clubs.

REFERENCES AND FURTHER READING

De Leon J, Bott A, Simpson GM. Dysmorphophobia: a body dysmorphic disorder or delusional disorder somatic subtype. *Comprehensive Psychiatry* 1989; 30(6): 457–72.

Frank DS. Dysmorphophobia. In: Gaind RN, Fawzy FI, Hudson BL, Pasnau RO. *Current Theories in Psychiatry*. New York: Medical and Scientific Books Vol 4, 1985.

Gelder M, Gath D, Mayou R eds. *Oxford Textbook of Psychiatry* (second edition). Oxford: Oxford University Press, 1989: Chapter 12 p 417–418.

Harris D. The benefits and hazards of cosmetic surgery. *British Journal of Hospital Medicine* 1989; 41: 540–45.

Rogers CR. *Client Centered Therapy: its Current Practice, Implications and Theory*. London: Constable, 1951.

---

1 A useful self-help book is: Dickinson A. *A Woman in Your Own Right*. London: Quartet, 1982.

QUESTION 16B

You are asked by the house officer in cardiology to see a very intense and ambitious 55 year old executive on a medical ward who had a myocardial infarction (MI) two weeks ago. He appears to be "depressed" and is not eating. How would you (a) go about assessing him and (b) treat him if he has a major depressive illness?

ANSWER 16B

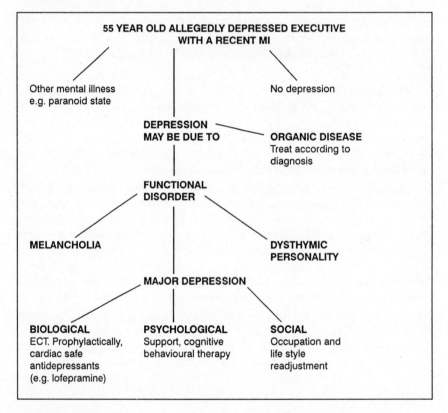

ASSESSMENT

General opening/special features of the case

My assessment will have to find out: whether the patient is depressed at all; if he has a major depressive illness[2] and how severe it is; by how much his depression is an understandable reaction to his illness

---

2 Major depressive disorder, melancholia and dysthymic personality are terms defined in the *Diagnosis and Statistical Manual of Mental Disorders* (3rd edition revised) (DSM-IIIR) Washington DC: American Psychiatric Association.

(melancholia)[2] or part of his personality (dysthymic personality)[2]; and whether organic factors may have either produced or mimicked the symptoms of the depression. I would also bear in mind that he may have some other mental illness masquerading as a depression.

Sources of history
I would need: his medical notes (including investigations); to interview the nurses looking after the patient and the patient himself. I would like to see his spouse or a close relative.

History and mental state examination

Biological
I would review the medical notes to exclude an organic basis to the depression – it would be essential to look for both the complications of MI (e.g. infection) and evidence of other physical disorders (e.g. hypothyroidism) which may have been inadvertently revealed by the investigations.

I would ask the nurse in charge of his care about his sleep, calorie and fluid intake, and weight. I would also be interested in: any abnormal ideas he may have been expressing, especially negative ideas about self, interpretation of experiences and expectations of the future (*Beck's triad*[3]) and assess his *suicidal intent*[4]; any change of behaviour (particularly of confusion or social withdrawal); how long he has been depressed and whether any activities or interests can lift his mood.

I would carefully examine his mental state not only for evidence of a depressive illness, but for evidence of any other mental disorder which may be masquerading as a depression (e.g. paranoid or alcohol withdrawal states). Because the *biological symptoms of depression*, such as poor energy and sleep disturbance, which point to a major depressive illness, may be indistinguishable from the effects of cardiac disease, I would base my assessment of the depression principally on the nature of his beliefs (e.g. marked hopelessness or suicidal ideas) and their duration (greater than two weeks), and on the cessation of vital bodily functions such as refusing to eat or drink, or failure to attend to matters of personal hygiene or elimination.

I would also bear in mind that the patient may have been prone to periods of low mood (*dysthymic personality*), or that he may not be depressed at all and, simply, obtaining some form of *secondary gain* through *abnormal illness behaviour*.

I would test his cognitive function to exclude an organic condition such as an acute confusional state.

---

3 Becks' triad, cross reference question 17A.
4 Suicidal intent, cross reference question 17A.

Psychological

Irrespective of whether he has a mental illness or not, the impact of the MI on his current life circumstances and expectations may be a source of considerable anxiety and introspection. For example, he may: have feelings of guilt or regret; worry about not being able to return to a "normal" life (concerns about a reduction in sexual performance are common); even have an existential "crisis" (i.e. a wish to re-think, or fundamentally alter the course of his life or beliefs). I would assess his personality particularly with regard to *type A features* (excessive ambition, hostility and a chronic sense of urgency).

Social

Practical issues will need to be addressed. Is he at risk of losing his job or status? Does his illness have financial repercussions (e.g. inadequate insurance cover)? Is he entitled to sickness or social security benefits (specialist advice would be sought via a social worker)?

TREATMENT

General opening/special features of the case

If he has a major depressive illness and has stopped eating, he will need rapid and effective treatment by the method with the least risk of aggravating his heart condition.

Biological

I would put the patient on a calorie, fluid balance and weight chart and regularly review it. In this acute situation, I would consider *electroconvulsive treatment (ECT)*. If maintenance or prophylactic treatment is indicated, I would wait until at least a month after his MI before starting him on an antidepressant with a low risk of *cardiotoxic side-effects* (e.g. *lofepramine*). Increments to his antidepressant dose should be gradual, and I would regularly monitor his pulse, blood pressure and electrocardiogram for evidence of cardiotoxicity such as tachycardia, marked hypotension or conduction disturbance.

Psychological

While he is receiving ECT and later, antidepressants, I would provide *supportive psychotherapy*. If, however, chronic stresses remain, or a change of personal style is advisable (to reduce type A behaviour and therefore, possibly, the risk of another MI), I would advise psychotherapy[5] aimed specifically at these problems such as *interpersonal*

---

5 Examiners can have strong views about psychotherapy. In this question, the author has stated his choice. Students are advised to mention a type of psychotherapy which they could discuss further with conviction.

psychotherapy. Coronary after-care groups (aimed at reducing type A behaviour) are helpful. I may also need to counsel his family in order to maximise their support for him and to allay, if possible, some of their own fears.

Social
This would be dependent on the amount of social or occupational change that is necessary.

REFERENCES AND FURTHER READING

Freeman CPL. Electroconvulsive therapy: its current clinical use. *British Journal of Hospital Medicine* March 1979; 281–292.

Friedman M, Thorensen CE, Gill JJ. Feasibility of alterating Type A behaviour after myocardial infarction. Recurrent coronary prevention project study: methods, base line results and preliminary findings. *Circulation* 1982; 66: 83–92.

Gelder M, Gath D, Mayor R. *Oxford Textbook of Psychiatry* (second edition). Oxford: Oxford University Press 1989: Chapter 8 p 217–223 and Chapter 176 679–89.

Mechanic D. *Medical Sociology* (second edition). Glencoe: Free Press, 1978.

Weissman M, Prusoff B, Di Mascio A et al. The efficacy of drugs and psychotherapy in the treatment of acute depressive episodes. *American Journal of Psychiatry* 1979; 136: 555–8.

CHAPTER 17

ASSESSMENT OF THE SUICIDAL PATIENT AND OF DELIBERATE SELF-HARM

QUESTION 17A

You are asked to see a 19 year old girl on the general medical ward who recently took an overdose of ten tablets (500 mg/tablet) of paracetamol with some alcohol. How would you assess her?

Although she has no obvious clinical symptoms, her blood tests show that she needs urgent treatment to prevent hepatic damage. She is, however, refusing all treatment. How would you advise the physicians to proceed?

ANSWER 17A

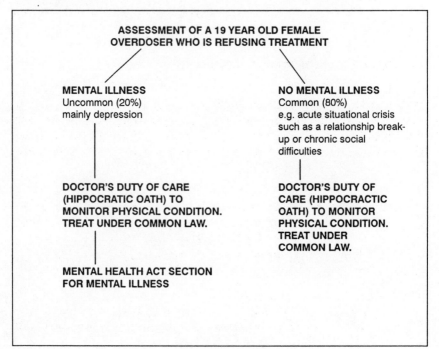

ASSESSMENT OF A 19 YEAR OLD FEMALE
OVERDOSER WHO IS REFUSING TREATMENT

MENTAL ILLNESS
Uncommon (20%)
mainly depression

NO MENTAL ILLNESS
Common (80%)
e.g. acute situational crisis
such as a relationship break-
up or chronic social
difficulties

DOCTOR'S DUTY OF CARE
(HIPPOCRATIC OATH) TO
MONITOR PHYSICAL CONDITION.
TREAT UNDER COMMON LAW.

DOCTOR'S DUTY OF
CARE (HIPPOCRACTIC
OATH) TO MONITOR
PHYSICAL CONDITION.
TREAT UNDER
COMMON LAW.

MENTAL HEALTH ACT SECTION
FOR MENTAL ILLNESS

ASSESSMENT

General opening/special features of the case

I would conduct the assessment to determine the patient's: immediate risk of suicide (*suicide intent*), risk of further deliberate self-harm; and any current medical or social problems.

I would ensure that my interview with her was conducted in a private place with the minimum risk of interruption (preferably, a side-room). I would also check that the patient was physically well enough to be interviewed, if not, I would arrange to return when she is. My style would be systematic, sympathetic, and non-judgemental or challenging, with every opportunity for her to put forward constructive solutions, either through self-help or with the aid of the facilities she could reasonably draw upon, to address any personal or social problems she may have.

Sources of history

Primarily the patient. It is, however, usually prudent to see a close relative or her partner if she has one. The nurses on the ward may be able to provide useful information about her physical state and her prevailing emotional condition (e.g. do visitors cheer her up, or has the arrival of a boyfriend or other family member "magically" resolved the situation?).

History and mental state examination

Biological
I would look for evidence of a current mental illness with special attention to *depression, personality disorder* and *alcohol misuse*, and take note of additional factors which increase the *risk of repetition* (e.g. previous attempts, a past psychiatric history, criminal record, low social class and unemployment).

Psychological
I would assess the patient's *suicidal intent*[1]. That is, was the act planned? Was there a final act (e.g. a suicide note)? Does the patient regret the overdose? Does she still wish to die?

I would look for current *life stresses* (interpersonal problems, and difficulties with loneliness, or low self-esteem are common).

Social
I would look in to, if they exist, what can practically be done about the social difficulties (e.g. these may include poor housing, receiving

---

1 See reference 1 for a scale to assess suicidal intent.

inadequate benefits, having to look after a young child?). The help of a social worker or social services may be needed.

MANAGEMENT OF TREATMENT REFUSAL

Every effort, including the help of someone she was close to, would be used to persuade her to accept treatment voluntarily. However, regardless of whether or not the patient had a mental illness, I would advise the physicians to monitor her clinical condition using non-invasive techniques (e.g. pulse, blood pressure, respiration, level of consciousness), because all doctors have a *duty of care* (under the *Hippocratic oath*) to their patients. If it becomes clear that life saving treatment is necessary, I would advise this to proceed under *common law*, especially if the patient's clinical condition is such that she can no longer give informed consent (e.g. she may be confused).

If the patient had a mental disorder, it would be appropriate to apply for her to be detained in hospital for assessment and treatment (Section 2 of the *Mental Health Act*).

REFERENCES AND FURTHER READING

Beck AT, Schuyler D, Herman I. Development of suicide intent scales. In: Beck AT, HLP Rasaik, DJ Lettie eds. *The Prediction of Suicide*. Maryland: Charles Press, 1974.

Gelder M, Gath D, Mayou R. *Oxford Textbook of Psychiatry* (second edition). Oxford: Oxford University Press, 1989: chapter 13 p 497–506.

Hawton KE, Catalan J. *Attempted Suicide: a Practical Guide to its Nature and Management* (second edition). Oxford: Oxford University Press, 1987.

Morgan HG. *Death Wishes?* Chichester: John Wiley Press & Sons Ltd, 1979.

Puxon M. Informed consent. *British Journal of Hospital Medicine* 1985; 34(1): 6.

QUESTION 17B

You have been asked to see a 19 year old nurse by her general practitioner because she has been making "superficial" cuts to her wrist since she split up with her boyfriend two weeks ago.
What would your management be?

ANSWER 17B

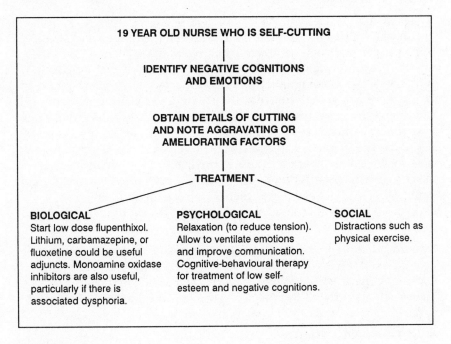

19 YEAR OLD NURSE WHO IS SELF-CUTTING

IDENTIFY NEGATIVE COGNITIONS AND EMOTIONS

OBTAIN DETAILS OF CUTTING AND NOTE AGGRAVATING OR AMELIORATING FACTORS

TREATMENT

BIOLOGICAL
Start low dose flupenthixol. Lithium, carbamazepine, or fluoxetine could be useful adjuncts. Monoamine oxidase inhibitors are also useful, particularly if there is associated dysphoria.

PSYCHOLOGICAL
Relaxation (to reduce tension). Allow to ventilate emotions and improve communication. Cognitive-behavioural therapy for treatment of low self-esteem and negative cognitions.

SOCIAL
Distractions such as physical exercise.

ASSESSMENT

General opening/special features of the case

The management of the *self-cutting* behaviour would be dependent on the assessment of the cognitions and emotions which produced it, and the development of strategies to reduce or abolish it.

Sources of history

I would interview the patient and, separately, a close friend or relative on whom she relies.

History and mental state examination

Biological
I would look for a family history of mental illness, an upbringing characterised by parental discord, separation or emotional aloofness

with little physical contact (particularly by the mother); she could volunteer evidence of physical or sexual abuse; and there could be a personal history of depression, mood swings, eating disorder, substance misuse or sexual dysfunction.

Additionally, I would exclude a psychotic disorder; this, however, is more common with deep lacerations or self-mutilations.

I would assess her risk of *deliberate self-harm* (e.g. by overdosing or self-cutting, and *suicide*).

Psychological
I would carry out a thorough *behavioural analysis* of the events leading up to the self-cutting – what were the precipitating events? Were there any negative cognitions (e.g. "I hate myself, I'm not worth anything")? What was the accompanying emotional tone (anger, low mood or tension are common)? How did the thoughts of cutting develop and was there any attempt to distract herself from them? Were there any associated behaviours (e.g. finding a place and/or an instrument)? What factors increased her likelihood of cutting (excessive drinking and social isolation are frequently reported)? How many cuts were made? How deep were they? Was there any pain (the absence of pain is usual) and afterwards, was there any relief of tension?

I would also look for evidence of low self-esteem or obsessionality.

Social
I would be interested in the reaction of her friends or relatives to the cutting – did it help her to get what she wanted (i.e. secondary gain)? Did they collude with it? Were they irritated or angered by it, and was she rejected by them? Did they offer the appropriate level of support?

Physical examination

I would examine her injuries, and organise appropriate medical treatment. Excessive scarring could require plastic surgery.

MANAGEMENT

General opening/special features of the case

I would ensure that she was motivated to give up her self-cutting before embarking on a management programme; the aims would be to assist her with reducing her cutting, and to resolve any underlying conflicts.

I would treat her as an out-patient. If in-patient treatment is indicated by overwhelming life crises or very frequent cutting, I would draw up a *limit-setting contract* between herself and the ward, and ensure that the staff were aware of their roles and prepared to maintain a consistent approach to her management.

Biological
I would start her on a low dose of a neuroleptic such as flupenthixol to reduce anxiety. Drugs which enhance brain 5HT function such as *lithium*, and *fluoxetine* would appear to be particularly beneficial. *Carbamazepine or a monoamine oxidase inhibitor* could also be used, especially if there was depressed mood.

Psychological
I would challenge the: negative cognitions associated with the cutting; low self-esteem; and the mood swings using a *cognitive-behavioural approach*. *Communication difficulties* and the *ventilation of emotions* (especially about the relationship break-up) would be addressed using role play. And, I would encourage her to attend a *relaxation class*.

Social
I would advise that she attempt to *channel her anxiety* in to a sport (e.g. swimming) or leisure activity. Alternatively, she could attempt more specific strategies such as squeezing a rubber ball until the discomfort causes her to stop.

REFERENCES AND FURTHER READING

Beck AT, Rush AJ, Shaw BF et al. *Cognitive Therapy of Depression*. New York: Guildford, 1979.

Hawton K. Self-cutting: can it be prevented. In: *Dilemmas and Difficulties in the Management of Psychiatric Patients*. Hawton K and Cowen P (editors).

Weissman MM. Wrist-cutting: relationship between clinical observations and epidemiological findings. *Archives of General Psychiatry* 1975; 32: 1166–71.

Winchel RM, Stanley M. Self injurious behaviour: a review of self mutilation. *American Journal of Psychiatry* (March) 1991: 306–17.

CHAPTER 18

SEASONAL AFFECTIVE DISORDER

QUESTION 18

You have been asked by a general practitioner to see a 24 year old woman who for the last three years has been depressed with hypersomnia and weight gain between the months of October and April. She spent most of last winter in Africa, and was not depressed, but in the spring became hypomanic characterized by mild elation, overactivity, and irritability.

What would your management be?

What is the underlying mechanism of her illness?

ANSWER 18

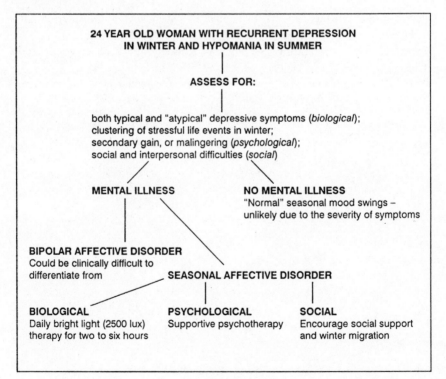

ASSESSMENT

General opening/special features of the case

Management would be dependent on assessment.

Although mood change, with dysthymia in winter and euthymia or mild elation in summer, is commonly reported by normal individuals, its extent, in this case, would suggest a pathological process – *seasonal affective disorder*. And because the mood change with season could be coincidental, the main differential diagnosis to exclude would be a *bipolar affective disorder*.

Sources of history

I would interview the patient, and separately, a reliable informant such as a relative or close friend.

History and mental state examination

Biological
I would be interested in the *onset, nature* and *progression of her symptoms*. While "*atypical depressive symptoms*" – hypersomnia, carbohydrate craving, bingeing, weight gain and irritability – starting in late autumn or winter followed by euthymia or hypomania in spring, would be characteristic of seasonal affective disorder; in the depressive phase of a bipolar affective disorder, *biological symptoms of depression* would be typical. Fatigue, loss of libido, menstrual irregularities and a family history of major affective disorder would be common to both.

As with all depressions, I would assess suicide risk[1].

Psychological
I would look for an excess of *stressful life events* during winter months. For instance, some occupations such as working for a charity for the elderly during a severe winter could be onerous. And, there could, coincidentally, be a cluster of adverse personal anniversaries (e.g. bereavements).

Evidence of secondary gain or malingering would be sought.

Social
I would explore the *quality of her interpersonal relationships* and *social life* – patients with seasonal affective disorder would be expected to report a greater difficulty to sustain relationships in winter compared with summer – the freedom from depression while in Africa could have been due to *escaping from an intolerable situational crisis at home*; alternatively, the southern migration (to Africa) could have been

---

1 Cross reference question 17a: assessment of suicide risk.

responsible for her clinical improvement by increasing her exposure to daylight.

MANAGEMENT

General opening/special features of the case

Seasonal affective disorder would be the most likely diagnosis; in clinical practice however, because of the mood swings, it could be difficult to distinguish from bipolar affective disorder.

Treatment would be on an outpatient basis.

Biological
The standard regime would be *bright light (2500 lux* for two to six hours per day)[2], delivered by a fluorescent box installed in the patient's home.

Psychological
I would offer her *supportive psychotherapy*; often, this has to commence before the manifestation of depressive symptoms in autumn to reduce anticipatory anxiety.

Social
I would help with *educating* her friends and family about the nature of her illness to foster their support.

Southern migration during winter would be encouraged.

MECHANISM OF ACTION

The mechanism for the antidepressant effect of light therapy is largely unknown: the time of day the treatment is administered is not crucial, and there is no convincing evidence that resynchronization of delayed nocturnal melatonin secretion is of aetiological significance.

REFERENCES AND FURTHER READING

Abas M, Murphy D. Seasonal affective disorder: the miseries of long dark nights? *British Medical Journal* 1987; 295: 1504–5.

Gelder M, Gath D, Mayou R. *Oxford Textbook of Psychiatry* (second edition). Oxford: Oxford University Press, 1989; chapter 8 p 230.

Lewy AJ, Sack RL, Miller S et al. Antidepressant and circadian phase-shifting effects of light. *Science* 1987; 235: 352–4.

Rosenthal NE, Sack DA, Gillin CJ et al. Seasonal affective disorder: a description of the syndrome and preliminary findings with light therapy. *Archives of General Psychiatry* 1984; 41: 72–80.

---

2 Dim light (<100 lux) is not effective in treating seasonal affective disorder.

CHAPTER 19

SCHOOL REFUSAL, ADOLESCENT SUICIDE, AND NON-ACCIDENTAL INJURY

QUESTION 19A

You have been asked by a general practitioner to see an 11 year old boy who is not attending school. His attendance at his last school was excellent, and his academic performance good.

How would you assess him?

What is the most likely diagnosis, and what would your treatment be?

ANSWER 19A

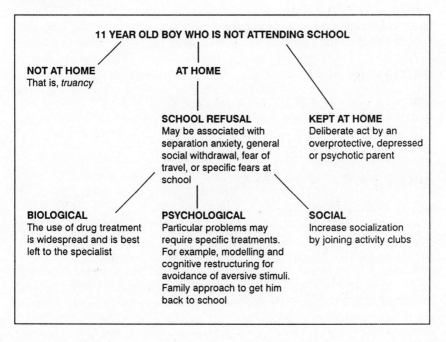

11 YEAR OLD BOY WHO IS NOT ATTENDING SCHOOL

NOT AT HOME
That is, *truancy*

AT HOME

SCHOOL REFUSAL
May be associated with separation anxiety, general social withdrawal, fear of travel, or specific fears at school

KEPT AT HOME
Deliberate act by an overprotective, depressed or psychotic parent

BIOLOGICAL
The use of drug treatment is widespread and is best left to the specialist

PSYCHOLOGICAL
Particular problems may require specific treatments. For example, modelling and cognitive restructuring for avoidance of aversive stimuli. Family approach to get him back to school

SOCIAL
Increase socialization by joining activity clubs

ASSESSMENT

General opening/special features of the case

The purpose of the assessment would be to determine whether he was absent from school and: not at home – *truanting*; at home – *school refusing*; or *deliberately kept at home* by one or both parents. Sometimes, there is a mixed picture of school refusal and truanting.

Sources of history

I would obtain a full developmental and psychiatric history of the boy from his parents, and visit the school to talk to his teachers and the educational psychologist. The boy's general practitioner would be contacted to obtain the details of his presenting complaint and the treatment he has received.

I would interview the boy on his own in a room containing a selection of age-appropriate toys, and with enough space to allow him to physically express himself. A family assessment would also be essential.

History and mental state examination

Biological

I would be interested in a family history of *depression* or *anxiety*. And I would determine the nature, onset, and progression of the boy's symptoms. That is, where was he, if not at school? If he was at home, did he have any somatic complaints? How did his parents react to his refusal to go to school? Were there any associated psychological symptoms? When did he last go to school?

Psychological

In the boy, I would look for: any *life events* such as a change of school, the departure of a significant person from his life or other separations which could be associated with irritability, anxiety or mood change; *generalised* or *specific fears* of travelling to and at school such as school size, sexual talk, particular lessons or games, bullying or punishment; *personality difficulties* which could include a *negative self-evaluation* or *low self-esteem*, stubbornness, resistance to pressure, and inability to persuade other family members, antisocial or delinquent behaviour. Furthermore, I would be interested in any evidence of obvious physical or sexual immaturity, or handicapping conditions. A full assessment of intellectual and academic attainment would be made.

I would explore the families' methods of coping with anxiety, death, separations or other life events and any parental threats (often by mother) to leave home or commit suicide as a way of expressing anger or controlling the boy. And I would assess the quality of his parent's relationship (e.g. were there any marital problems and how was power shared in the family?) and their psychological health (e.g. the boy could have been overprotected, or deliberately kept at home by a depressed or psychotic parent).

Social
I would ascertain the boy's level of social functioning both with and without the family set up, and evaluate his parents' attitudes to education and their commitment to get him back to school.

Physical examination

An appropriate medical and neurological examination would be undertaken.

MANAGEMENT

General opening/special features of the case

The most likely diagnosis is school refusal.

The management aim would be to return the boy to school as quickly as possible. The four steps would be to: establish a therapeutic relationship with the boy and his family; identify the stimuli or situations which give rise to anxiety at home or at school; choose the appropriate method of desensitizing the boy to the feared situation; confront the feared situation. Although treatment would be on an outpatient basis, day or in-patient *milieu therapy* would be appropriate if this did not succeed.

It would also be necessary for me to liaise with the school to organize an educational programme: some schools, particularly in inner city areas, have special units within the school for the educationally disaffected children and hold special tutorial sessions designed to help such children catch up educationally. Home tuition could increase the boy's social isolation, and in itself, should not be a treatment programme.

Biological
The use of antidepressant or other drug treatments[1] is not currently widespread and is, perhaps, best left to the specialist.

Psychological
Particular problems could require specific treatments. For example, appropriate treatments for excessive fearfulness/generalised anxiety,

---

1 Imipramine, a tricyclic antidepressant, may be helpful in the management of school refusal; its mechanism of action is, however, not related to its antidepressant activity. Other drugs such as alprazolam have also been reported to be of benefit.

avoidance of aversive social situations, attention-seeking behaviour, separation anxiety, or parental reinforcement of the behaviour would include desensitization/relaxation training, modelling and cognitive restructuring, shaping and differential reinforcement of other behaviour and contingency contracting for each condition respectively.

A family approach to getting the boy to school would be adopted. If the parents were up to it, they would be encouraged to take the boy to school on the first day. It would be particularly important for me to be in regular contact with the parents and to provide support during the first fortnight of reinstating the boy at school. Thereafter, reviews of progress and advice on recognizing high-risk situations for relapse (e.g. illness in the boy necessitating a prolonged period away from school, the start of a new term, or family illness or bereavement) would be carried out at appropriate intervals. More formal *family therapy* or *individual psychotherapy* could be needed.

Social
Improving peer relationships by joining activity clubs would be encouraged.

REFERENCES AND FURTHER READING

Bernstein GA, Garfinkel BD, Borchardt CM. Comparative studies of pharmacotherapy for school refusal. *Journal of the American Academy of Child and Adolescent Psychiatry* 1990; 29(5): 773–81.

Gelder M, Gath D, Mayou R. *Oxford Textbook of Psychiatry* (second edition). Oxford: Oxford University Press 1989; chapter 20 p 787–9.

Kearney CA, Silverman WK. A preliminary analysis of a functional model of assessment and treatment for school refusal behavior. *Behavior Modification* 1990; 14(3): 340-66.

Rutter ML, Hersov L. *Child and Adolescent Psychiatry. Modern Approaches* Oxford: Blackwell, 1985.

Watters J. School refusal. *British Medical Journal* 1989; 298: 66–7.

QUESTION 19B

You have been asked to see a 13 year old boy who has "accidentally" swallowed 20 tablets of paracetamol.

How would you assess him?

ANSWER 19B

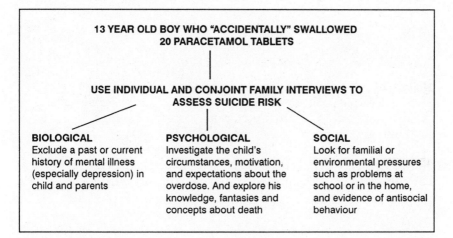

ASSESSMENT

General opening/special features of the case

I would take the overdose of paracetamol seriously and assess him for suicidal risk[2]. A detailed history from the child and his family would be used to: assess the child's suicidal tendencies and the conditions that increase the risk of suicidal behaviour; appraise the risk of repetition (short and long term); evaluate the child's emotional state, behaviours and interpersonal relationships.

It would also be important to establish a good therapeutic relationship with the child and to obtain his agreement to desist from further episodes of deliberate self-harm.

Sources of history

At first I would interview the child and his family individually, and subsequently, together.

The interview with the child would be conducted verbally at an appropriate level; this would emphasize the gravity of the situation and signal to the child that intense feelings or impulses should be

---

2 For a description of scales devised to assess suicidal risk such as the Child Suicide Potential scale see Pfeffer 1986.

openly discussed to find alternative ways of coping (rather than acting out suicidal impulses). Additionally, an open and frank discussion would render ineffective any covert threats the child could be planning to use to manipulate me.

A *problem-solving* approach during family interview would be used to recognise and help with any problems of communication, conflict resolution or power sharing associated with the suicidal behaviour.

History and mental state

There are *ten* areas of inquiry.

Biological
Firstly, I would look for a *parental history of depression*, substance misuse, completed or attempted suicide, and emotional deprivation in childhood.

Secondly, in the child, I would be interested in any *previous or current evidence of psychopathology*: particularly depression (biological symptoms could be present), anxiety, temper tantrums, psychosis or fire setting.

Psychological
Thirdly, I would find out what the child's circumstances were at the time of the overdose – for examples, what was he doing? What was his prevailing mood? Was he alone or with others? Did he warn anyone? Had he consumed any alcohol? Did he leave a suicide note?

Fourthly, I would look for any factors which could have motivated the child's overdose – examples include rejection (usually by a girlfriend), revenge at someone who hurt him, a cry for help, a wish to contact a dead loved person, an exploratory gamble to test whether someone loves him, identification with a cult figure, or manipulative or attention seeking behaviour.

Fifthly, I would ascertain what the child thought the consequences of the overdose would be.

Sixthly, I would assess the child's experience of suicidal behaviour – for examples, had he thought or attempted to kill himself before? Did he know anyone who had attempted or succeeded at committing suicide ? What method did that person use, when did it happen, and did he know whether the person had wished to die? How did he feel at the time?

Seventhly, I would establish what the child's fantasies about suicide were.

Eighthly, I would explore the child's thoughts and fantasies about death – for examples, did he think people went to a better place after death or could come back to life? Did he frequently think about death? What feelings did he have towards his own death?

Social
Ninthly, I would investigate whether the child was experiencing any intolerable familial or environmental situations from which he wished to temporarily or permanently escape – examples include bullying, poor achievement or relationships at school, or excessive discipline or abuse at home.

Finally, I would be interested in any evidence of *assaultive or antisocial behaviour*, or social maladjustment.

REFERENCES AND FURTHER READING

Haim A. *Adolescent Suicide*. Norfolk: Tavistock Publications, 1974.

Pfeffer CE. *The Suicidal Child*. New York: Guilford Press, 1986.

Rutter M. The developmental psychopathology of depression: issues and perspectives. *In: Rutter M, Izard CE, Read PB (editors). Depression in Young People: Developmental and Clinical Perspectives*. New York: Guilford Press, 1986.

Taylor EA, Stansfeld SA. Children who poison themselves: A clinical comparison with psychiatric controls. *British Journal of Psychiatry* 1984a; 145: 127-31.

Teicher J. A solution to the chronic problem of living: adolescent attempted suicide. *In Current Issues of Adolescent Psychiatry*, Schoolar J (editor). New York: Brunner Mozelh.

Cross reference Question 17a

QUESTION 19C

While attached to the accident and emergency department as a liaison psychiatrist, you are approached by a junior doctor who has recently seen a nine year old boy for bruises to his upper body, and fractures to his right femur and head. He recalls that he has treated the boy on at least three other occasions in the last six months for bruises to his thigh and a fracture to his left collar bone. The boy's parents are reluctant to discuss the details of the injuries. The junior doctor is suspicious that the boy is being physically abused by his parents but does not know what to do next.

How should the junior doctor proceed?

How should the paediatricians proceed, and what are the important aspects of the assessment of the boy and his family?

ANSWER 19C

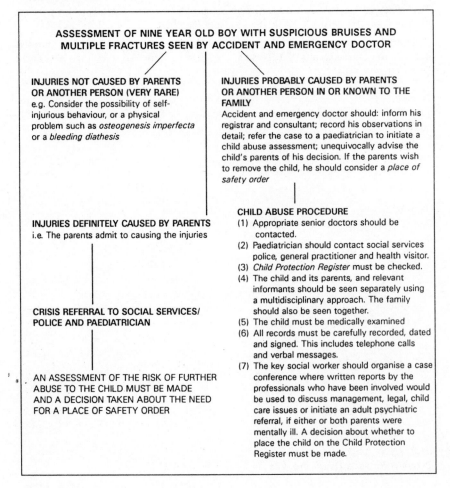

ASSESSMENT OF NINE YEAR OLD BOY WITH SUSPICIOUS BRUISES AND MULTIPLE FRACTURES SEEN BY ACCIDENT AND EMERGENCY DOCTOR

INJURIES NOT CAUSED BY PARENTS OR ANOTHER PERSON (VERY RARE)
e.g. Consider the possibility of self-injurious behaviour, or a physical problem such as *osteogenesis imperfecta* or a *bleeding diathesis*

INJURIES PROBABLY CAUSED BY PARENTS OR ANOTHER PERSON IN OR KNOWN TO THE FAMILY
Accident and emergency doctor should: inform his registrar and consultant; record his observations in detail; refer the case to a paediatrician to initiate a child abuse assessment; unequivocally advise the child's parents of his decision. If the parents wish to remove the child, he should consider a *place of safety order*

INJURIES DEFINITELY CAUSED BY PARENTS
i.e. The parents admit to causing the injuries

CRISIS REFERRAL TO SOCIAL SERVICES/ POLICE AND PAEDIATRICIAN

AN ASSESSMENT OF THE RISK OF FURTHER ABUSE TO THE CHILD MUST BE MADE AND A DECISION TAKEN ABOUT THE NEED FOR A PLACE OF SAFETY ORDER

CHILD ABUSE PROCEDURE
(1) Appropriate senior doctors should be contacted.
(2) Paediatrician should contact social services police, general practitioner and health visitor.
(3) *Child Protection Register* must be checked.
(4) The child and its parents, and relevant informants should be seen separately using a multidisciplinary approach. The family should also be seen together.
(5) The child must be medically examined
(6) All records must be carefully recorded, dated and signed. This includes telephone calls and verbal messages.
(7) The key social worker should organise a case conference where written reports by the professionals who have been involved would be used to discuss management, legal, child care issues or initiate an adult psychiatric referral, if either or both parents were mentally ill. A decision about whether to place the child on the Child Protection Register must be made.

General opening/special features of the case

The child's repeated and unexplained fractures and bruises could be due to physical abuse by one or both parents. It would, however, be essential to consider that the abuse could have been carried out by someone other than the parents who is about at home (e.g. an older sibling) or someone who visits the home regularly (e.g. friends or relatives). And I would be mindful that the child could also have been abused in other ways, for example, sexually.

The *statutory obligation* to investigate all suspected cases of child physical abuse, although subject to local[3] variations, is the responsibility of the Social Services and/or the police. From the outset, it would be important to establish a satisfactory working relationship with the parents which would facilitate effective future supervision and management; this, however, could be difficult to achieve especially if the parents were guarded, guilt-ridden, or over-anxious. A *non-judgemental approach* would be essential. *Stressing concern* for the child and the need to prevent further harm by exploring ways of helping the parents to find non-abusing ways of coping would be helpful. It would be important to assess: the safety and welfare of the child and the other children in the family (especially the risk of further abuse); the families needs; the evidence which could be used in legal (and criminal) proceedings against the parents and/or the responsible person. Furthermore, it would be crucial to look for non-abuse explanations for the injuries.

If, however, the child's parents openly admit to the abuse, a crisis referral should be made to the appropriate agencies – Social Services/Police and the paediatricians – who must decide on the need for a *place of safety order*.

[4]*Procedures to be followed in cases of probable child physical abuse by junior doctor in accident and emergency*

1. The junior doctor should inform his registrar, who should initiate the referral to the paediatric department (consultant or registrar on-call), and the accident and emergency consultant. The junior doctor should not undertake any further child abuse investigations.

2. The junior doctor should make a detailed record of the history

---

3 All clinicians should be acquainted with their local guidelines for assessing child abuse. These guidelines may alter with future amendments to the *Child Protection Act*.

4 Although the details would, of course, be different, the framework for investigating child physical and sexual abuse are similar.

and all his findings on examination. All records must be fully dated and signed.

3.   The junior doctor should clearly inform the child's parents that he would be requesting an investigation for child abuse, and that the child must be admitted to hospital for this purpose.

4.   If an attempt is made by the parents to remove the child from hospital, a place of safety order should be considered.

In cases of probable child physical abuse procedures to be followed by the paediatrician

1.   With the child in hospital, the consultant paediatrician (or in his absence the paediatric registrar) must immediately inform the on-call social worker (or the ward social worker if the referral was made during the day) and the police. The need for a place of safety order should be discussed.

2.   The appropriate Paediatric Medical Social Worker and Principal Officer (Social Services) must be informed and asked for any information known to them about the family (especially prior enrolment on the *Child Protection Register*).

3.   The general practitioner and health visitor (if one has been allocated) must be informed; they should be, specifically, asked about the child's previous state of health, development, behaviour and injuries (including any action taken. Any information on the physical, and mental health of the child's parents and relevant details of other siblings (e.g. unexplained injuries) and of the families' living conditions (including people who shared or visited the home regularly) would be important.

4.   A *multidisciplinary interview* usually by the consultant paediatrician and the key social worker, of the child and its parents (at first separately, and subsequently together), and of any relevant informants must be undertaken and carefully recorded. The child would also need a detailed physical examination. All telephone or verbal communications should be written down. Information from the assessment would form the basis of written reports for a case conference organised by the key social worker. And all the professionals who have been involved with the assessment should be invited to the conference the purpose of which would be to discuss future management, legal or child care issues or the involvement of the adult psychiatric services if one or both parents was mentally ill.

IMPORTANT ASPECTS OF THE ASSESSMENT

Biological
In the child's parents, I would look for a history of mental illness (especially depression or psychosis), subnormality, or substance misuse, and for any chronic or recurrent medical problems, or cot deaths in the family.

In the child, I would look for evidence of unexplained failure to thrive or marked weight loss and consider the very rare but important possibilities that the injuries could have been due to self-injurious behaviour or caused by an underlying physical disorder such as *osteogenesis imperfecta or a bleeding diathesis.*

Psychological
In the child's parents, I would be interested in any evidence of violence in their own upbringing, separation or loss experiences in childhood (particularly if they have been in care), emotional problems or behavioural difficulties in childhood, serious physical or emotional deprivations in childhood, adverse reactions to stress, low self-esteem, and any difficulties associated with being parents in early adulthood.

I would look for any factors which could have contributed to his being a "*vulnerable child*" – being the product of an unwelcome or difficult pregnancy, a period of admission to a special care baby unit shortly after birth, other enforced separations within the first year of life, continuing medical problems, handicaps (physical or mental) or developmental delays, temperamental difficulty (especially where the parents are unable to copy with this stress) and unrealistic expectations of a psycho-social or academic nature. I would also look for *secondary behavioural* changes which could be associated with the abuse such as truancy, antisocial tendencies or difficulties with establishing peer relationships at school and "*frozen watchfulness*" or "*gaze avoidance*" when his parents are in the room.

Social
In the family, I would explore any financial stresses, lack of social support, and interpersonal or marital conflicts.

Physical examination

Although this would usually be co-ordinated by the paediatrician, other medical or surgical specialities could become involved.

A full physical and neurological investigation would be essential. In particular, all bruises and injuries must be mapped, and recorded according to type, site, size, number and resolution. Colour photographs would be of great benefit. The fundi should be examined. All findings must be accurately recorded, dated, and signed. An opinion should be given about the likelihood of the injuries being the result of physical or sexual abuse, or both.

Other important investigations would include a skeletal survey and a haematological profile (full blood count and film, platelets, and a full clotting screen).

REFERENCES AND FURTHER READING

Franklin AW. *Child Abuse*. Edinburgh: Churchill Livingstone, 1977.

Gelder M, Gath D, Mayou R. *Oxford Textbook of Psychiatry* (second edition) Oxford: Oxford University Press, 1989: chapter 20 p 809–14.

Minuchin S, Fishman HC. *Family Therapy Techniques*. Cambridge Massachusetts: Harvard University Press, 1981.

Oxfordshire area: *Child Protection Committee Procedures*.

Taitz LS. Child abuse and metabolic bone disease: are they often confused? *British Medical Journal* 1991; 302: 1244.

Wells C, Staurt I. *Self Destructive Behaviour in Children*. New York: Van Nostrand, Reinhold, 1981.

CHAPTER 20
EATING DISORDERS

QUESTION 20A

You are asked by the General Practitioner to arrange treatment for a 24 year old woman with a past history of Anorexia Nervosa who is rapidly losing weight and vomiting twice a day. At present, she is 5ft 7 inches (170 cm) tall and weighs 4½ stone (32.3 kg). The girl has lived with her mother all her life and they are said to go "everywhere together". The girl's mother separated from her father shortly before she was born.

How would you manage this situation?

ANSWER 20A

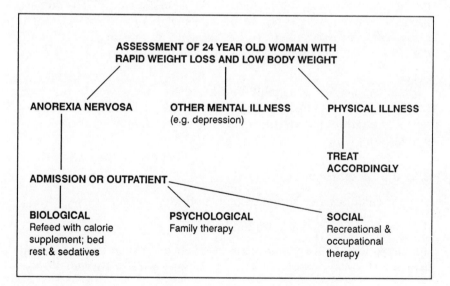

ASSESSMENT

General opening/special features of the case

Management of this situation is dependent on the assessment of the reason, onset and progression of the low body weight.

Sources of history

In their home, I would initially interview the girl and her mother separately and subsequently together. Next, it would be crucial to obtain information from other involved professionals e.g. the general practitioner and informants as well as referring to available medical or psychiatric case records.

History and mental state examination

Biological
I would be interested in the girl's: current pattern of eating (including binge-eating); rate of weight loss; menstrual history and behaviour directed towards weight loss e.g. excessive exercise and the use of diuretics or laxatives. I would look for a current, past or family history of mental illness, and enquire about her bowel habits.

Psychosocial
I would be interested in her attitudes towards body weight and shape. I would look specifically for evidence of low self-esteem, affective or psychotic disorder. During my observation of how the girl and her mother communicated and shared decisions, I would look for any proof of *enmeshment, overprotectiveness, rigidity* and *lack of conflict resolution.*[1] An assessment of her personality and in particular the stability of her personal relationships would be essential.

Social
I would explore the possibility that her drive to lose weight had been triggered by her occupation e.g. as in a ballet dancer, encouraged by peers or maintained by the response of her family to the "illness" (*secondary gain*).

Physical examination

I would calculate her *body mass index* (BMI)
$$\{BMI = \frac{weight\ (kg)}{height^2\ (m)}; 18\ is\ underweight\}$$
and look for signs of malnutrition such as oedema, dehydration, bradycardia, constipation, and low blood pressure, or thyroid disease.

Investigations

I would do: a full blood count to look for evidence of anaemia, infection, or metastatic disease; urea and electrolytes to assess the level of

---

1 For a description of how families may show enmeshment, overprotectiveness, rigidity and lack of conflict resolution see Minuchin S et al., 1978.

dehydration and to check for hypokalaemic acidosis and a thyroid function test to exclude thyroid disease.

Differential diagnosis/diagnostic formulation

The most likely diagnosis is of *anorexia nervosa* complicated by an overinvolved relationship with her mother.

The other possibilities are:

(a) anorexia nervosa complicated by mental illness e.g. depressive illness.

(b) Other mental disorders e.g. depressive illness or schizophrenia.

(c) Physical illness e.g. metastatic or thyroid disease, or rarely, tuberculosis.

MANAGEMENT

General opening/special features of the case

Anorexia nervosa is usually treated on an outpatient basis. In this case, however, her rapid weight loss would argue in favour of hospital admission.

Biological
I would start by trying to win her confidence by jointly setting a target weight (the weight or BMI can be used as a guide). Next, I would place her on bed rest and commence a programme of *refeeding* with an intake of 2,500–3,000 calories/day; it is sometimes necessary to administer a sedative dopamine receptor antagonist such as thioridazine to facilitate bed rest. In the first few weeks of refeeding I would build up the bulk content of the food gradually and use high calorie drinks. I would arrange for her toileting and meals to be supervised.

Psychosocial
She would be given *supportive psychotherapy* by her key workers. I would draw up, with the help of the psychologist, a behavioural programme based on the principle of providing simple rewards e.g. allowing her to have visitors in exchange for weight gain. Once her target weight is reached, and if they are willing, I would engage the girl and her mother in *family therapy*.

Social
I would encourage the girl to develop some independence and provide her with information on local self-help groups. The occupational therapist would be asked to assess her work skills and to provide remedial help if possible. The social worker would also be asked to assist with her rehabilitation back in to the community.

REFERENCES AND FURTHER READING

Gelder M, Gath D, Mayou R eds. *Oxford Textbook of Psychiatry* (2nd edition). Oxford: Oxford University Press, 1989: Chapter 12 p 436–42.

Garner DM, Garfinkel PE. *Handbook of Psychotherapy for Anorexia Nervosa and Bulimia*. New York: Guilford Press, 1985.

Minuchin S, Rosman B and Baker L. *Psychosomatic Families: Anorexia Nervosa in Context*. Cambridge, Mass: Harvard University Press, 1978.

Russel G F M. The current treatment of anorexia nervosa. *British Journal of Psychiatry* 1981; 138: 164–6.

QUESTION 20B

You have been asked to see a 21 year old air hostess by her general practitioner because she has been demanding slimming tablets to lose weight. Despite being only slightly underweight, she has admitted to drastic weight reduction measures. Often, she induces vomiting after "midnight feasts" to relieve the boredom of long haul flights, and fears that she has lost control over her eating. Her self-confidence is poor.
What would your management be?

ANSWER 20B

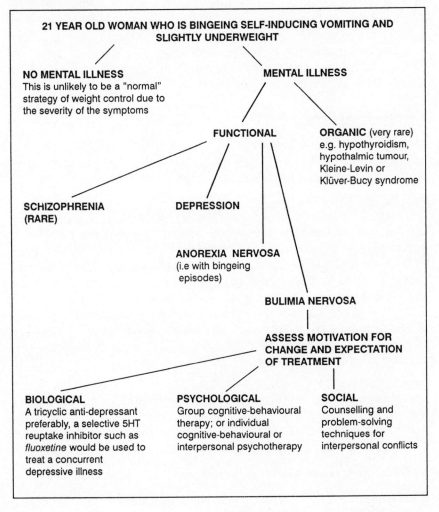

ASSESSMENT

General opening/special features of the case

Management would be dependent on assessment, the purpose of which would be to determine whether the episodes of bingeing are a secondary symptom of a functional disorder - for examples, anorexia nervosa[2], depression, borderline personality disorder, or, rarely, a psychosis (e.g. schizophrenia) – or, very rarely, due to an organic condition such as hypothyroidism, hypothalmic tumour, Klüver-Bucy or the Kleine-Levin syndrome); bingeing could also be the core symptom of a functional psychological disorder (i.e. *bulimia nervosa*). Furthermore, an unknown, but perhaps significant proportion of young women go through mild phases of self-induced vomiting after bingeing in an attempt to control their weight.

I would also assess her motivation to change the behaviour, and ensure that her expectations of treatment were not unrealistic.

Sources of history

I would interview the patient.[3]

History and mental state examination

Biological
I would be interested in a family history of *obesity, depression,* or *alcohol misuse,* and in the *onset, nature and progression of her symptoms.* Particular attention would be paid to: previous attempts at both normal and severe dietary control (a past history of anorexia nervosa would be important); obtaining a longitudinal record of her weight and calorie intake (a diary could be available) including the frequency of the binge-vomit cycles; uncovering dangerous methods of maintaining a low weight such as excessive exercise, or the misuse of laxatives or diuretics; menstrual irregularities; and any proof of a concurrent *depressive illness.*

Psychological
I would specifically look for evidence of: stressful *life events* such as the break up of a relationship, which could have triggered the behaviour; low self-esteem; negative attitudes towards her weight and

---

2 Up to 50% of patients with bulimia nervosa have a past history of anorexia nervosa. And, a small minority of patients meet the diagnostic criteria for both disorders.

3 Because the patient's behaviour may have been successfully concealed or considerable guilt or shame attached to it, the request to involve a partner or members of the family in the diagnostic or treatment process could be met with resistance.

shape (e.g. "I am too fat"); and poor impulse control such as hyper-sexuality, substance misuse, or repeated episodes of deliberate self-harm which could be associated with a *borderline personality disorder*.[4]

Social
I would assess how her lifestyle contributes to her bingeing – for example, there could be few opportunities to make and sustain interpersonal relationships, or the unusual hours of work could make normal dieting difficult.

Physical examination

I would conduct a thorough physical[5] and neurological examination (evidence of visual agnosia, raised intracranial pressure or stereo-typies would be significant), calculate her body mass index[6], and check her urea and electrolytes and thyroid function test for evidence of hypokalaemic alkalosis, hyponatraemia, or hypothyroidism respectively.

MANAGEMENT

General opening/special features of the case

The principles of managing bulimia nervosa include reducing the frequency of the binge-vomit cycle, helping the patient to gain control over her eating, challenging negative cognitive attitudes (especially low self-esteem), and treating any concurrent mental illness.

Biological
The request for slimming tablets would be tactfully but firmly declined.

---

4 A small but significant minority (in terms of treatment-resistance) of bulimic patients meet the diagnostic criteria for borderline personality disorder.
5 Bulimics often have a range of physical abnormalities such as enlargement of the parotid glands or toothache due to the erosion of the dental enamel, and minor biochemical disturbances (e.g. hyponatraemia, metabolic alkalosis, and hypokalaemia) which do not usually require specific treatment.
6 Body Mass Index: *Cross reference question 20A.*

If there was a concurrent depressive illness, I would prescribe a tricyclic antidepressant[7] (and in particular a selective 5HT reuptake inhibitor such as *fluoxetine*).

Psychological

My treatment of choice would be focal (approximately ten weeks in duration) *cognitive-behavioural group therapy* consisting of education (e.g. about diet plans), self monitoring (e.g. weight records), goal setting, assertiveness training, relaxation, and cognitive restructuring – to challenge distortions of body image, low mood, and find distractions to avoid bingeing urges; alternatives include cognitive-behavioural therapy on an individual basis or some other specific focal psychotherapy such as *interpersonal psychotherapy*.

Social

Counselling and problem-solving techniques would be a useful approach to resolving interpersonal conflicts.

A change of occupation to one she finds more stimulating should be considered.

REFERENCES AND FURTHER READING

Fairburn C. Bulimia nervosa. *British Medical Journal* 1990; 300: 485–7.

Freeman CLP, Barry F, Dunkeld-Turnbull J et al. Controlled trial of psychotherapy for bulimia nervosa. *British Medical Journal* 1988; 296: 521–5.

Gelder M, Gath D, Mayou R. *Oxford Textbook of Psychiatry* (second edition). Oxford: Oxford University Press, 1989; chapter 12 442–4.

Mynors-Wallis LM. The psychological treatment of eating disorders. *British Journal of Hospital Medicine* 1989; 41: 470–5.

---

7 The mechanism by which tricyclic antidepressants transiently reduce the intensity of bulimic symptoms is unknown, but it is probably independent of their antidepressant action; the reduction achieved by antidepressants compares favourably with the results of cognitive behavioural therapy. There is no added clinical benefit to combining antidepressant treatment with cognitive behavioural therapy. Selective 5HT reuptake inhibitors could be of additional value in the treatment of bulimia complicated by depression because they are less likely than first generation tricyclics to produce weight gain – a factor which can reduce the patient's compliance.

CHAPTER 21
PANIC DISORDER

QUESTION 21

You have been asked by a general practitioner to see a 22 year old University student who has recently developed panic attacks which occur up to three times a day. She is in her final year, and has recently broken up with her boyfriend. At the interview, she starts to have one of her attacks.

How would you treat this acute situation?

What would your management plan be?

ANSWER 21

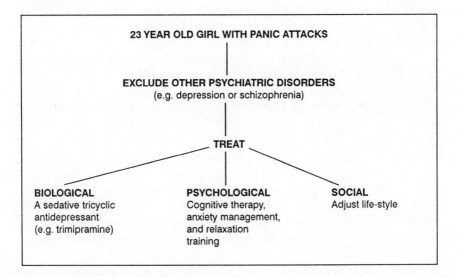

23 YEAR OLD GIRL WITH PANIC ATTACKS

EXCLUDE OTHER PSYCHIATRIC DISORDERS
(e.g. depression or schizophrenia)

TREAT

BIOLOGICAL
A sedative tricyclic antidepressant (e.g. trimipramine)

PSYCHOLOGICAL
Cognitive therapy, anxiety management, and relaxation training

SOCIAL
Adjust life-style

ACUTE TREATMENT OF THE PANIC ATTACK

I would: *firstly*, assure her that she would recover from the attack, and that she was not going to die;

secondly, tell her not to fight the panic, but to accept it;

thirdly, ask her to concentrate on breathing slowly, and supply her with a paper bag to breathe into;

fourthly, wait patiently for the attack to subside; and *fifthly*, reinforce her success.

ASSESSMENT

General opening/special features of the case

My management plan will depend on the assessment, the purpose of which would be to look for the cause of the panic attacks, and to ascertain what her coping strategies have been.

Sources of history

I would interview the patient, and any reliable informants. Also, it could prove necessary for me, with her permission, to talk to her tutors, especially if her examinations had to be rescheduled or postponed.

History and mental state examination

Biological

I would be interested in a family or personal history of mental illness, especially of *panic disorder*, a *generalised anxiety state, or depression*, and look for evidence of an associated functional (usually *depression*, although mania and schizophrenia would be important to exclude), or organic mental illness (see physical examination).

I would note any other distressing symptoms of anxiety, apart from those of panic, such as insomnia, restlessness, or appetite disturbance.

Psychological

While assessing the onset and progression of her symptoms, particular attention would be paid to both anticipated or recent *life events*, her anxieties about final examinations and the break of the relationship with her boyfriend. And I would be interested in uncovering any *dangerous coping strategies* such as *excessive alcohol consumption*, or drug misuse. I would look for evidence of reinforcing or maintaining factors.

I would assess her personality, primarily to determine whether she has always been an anxious person.

Social

I would find out what the attitude of her friends and family had been to her illness – were they supportive or was the illness encouraged in any way? – and evaluate the impact of her illness on her studies.

Physical examination

I would exclude organic causes of anxiety such as *thyrotoxicosis*, an *adrenal tumour*, and *hypoglycaemia*; thus, the cardiovascular system would be examined for tachycardia, atrial fibrillation and increased blood pressure, the eyes for exophthalmos and lid lag, and the nervous system for a fine non-intention tremor. Tests of thyroid function, a random blood glucose, and a full blood count would be done. Specific urine analysis for the breakdown products of catecholamine metabolism would only be carried out if there was a clear clinical indication for it.

MANAGEMENT

The management of *panic disorder* is dependent on whether or not a cause, at which treatment could be directed, had been identified.

If there was no obvious cause, the following plan would be carried out.

Biological
I would reduce the patient's symptoms[1] of anxiety with a tricyclic antidepressant with sedative and anxiolytic properties such as *trimipramine*; alternatively, *monoamine oxidase inhibitors* could be considered.

Benzodiazepines would be avoided because of the risk of dependence.

Psychological
Due to the high frequency of the panic attacks, I would undertake cognitive techniques such as thought stopping or voluntary hyperventilation; this could be more beneficial than *relaxation training* and *anxiety management classes* on their own.

Social
I would stress the importance of maintaining as normal a life-style as possible, getting the support of friends and relatives, and self-help through homework exercises she could carry out on her own to confront the fear.

REFERENCES AND FURTHER READING

Clark DM, Salkovskis PM, Chalkley AJ. Respiratory control as a treatment for panic attacks. *Journal of Behaviour Therapy and Experimental Psychiatry* 1985; 16: 23-30.

Gelder M, Gath D, Mayou R. *Oxford Textbook of Psychiatry* (second edition). Oxford: Oxford University Press, 1989; chapter 7 p 175-82.

Marks I. Behavioural psychotherapy in general psychiatry: helping patients to help themselves. *British Journal of Psychiatry* 1987; 150: 593-7.

---

1 Beta blockers are ineffective in the treatment of panic disorder.

Swinn R, Richardson F. Anxiety management training: a non-specific *behaviour therapy* programme for anxiety control. *Behaviour Therapy* 1971; 2: 498–510.

Tyrer P. Treating panic. *British Medical Journal* 1989; 298: 201.

CHAPTER 22

SELF-INJURIOUS BEHAVIOUR

QUESTION 22

A 14 year old boy who is mentally retarded is brought to you by his mother. For the last six months he has been banging his head, pinching and scratching himself repeatedly and his arms and legs are covered with scars and recent injuries. She has been unable to stop this behaviour. It has resulted in her having to spend more time with him, which is difficult as she has recently divorced and needs to work full-time.

How would you assess him?

How would you manage his behaviour if it was not due to mental illness?

ANSWER 22

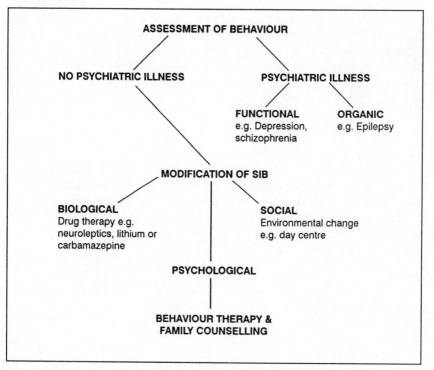

ASSESSMENT OF BEHAVIOUR

NO PSYCHIATRIC ILLNESS

PSYCHIATRIC ILLNESS

FUNCTIONAL
e.g. Depression,
schizophrenia

ORGANIC
e.g. Epilepsy

MODIFICATION OF SIB

BIOLOGICAL
Drug therapy e.g.
neuroleptics, lithium or
carbamazepine

SOCIAL
Environmental change
e.g. day centre

PSYCHOLOGICAL

BEHAVIOUR THERAPY &
FAMILY COUNSELLING

ASSESSMENT

General opening/special features of the case

Management is dependent on the assessment of the onset, nature and progression of the *self-injurious behaviour (SIB)* and its effect on his family.

Sources of history

In their home, I would initially interview the boy and his family separately and subsequently together. Next, it would be important to obtain information from other involved professionals e.g. teachers, social worker, school psychologist and general practitioner as well as referring to available medical or psychiatric case records.

History and mental state examination

Biological

I would be interested in any recent physical illness in the boy, the nature and extent of damage to property and of personal injury to all members of the family.

I would look for evidence of mental illness, particularly of *depression* (which may manifest as sadness, disturbance of appetite and sleep, or agitation), and *schizophrenia*[1] (although delusions or hallucinations may be difficult to elicit, there could be a change of mannerisms or stereotypies).

I would test his cognitive function for proof of organic impairment: and specifically enquire for *epilepsy*. If he is epileptic, I would ensure he was receiving the appropriate anticonvulsants in the therapeutic range, and had no evidence of drug toxicity.

Psychological

I would look for any evidence of: emotional stress (e.g. the departure of someone he was close to); pubertal problems; intellectual deterioration or of current, past or familial mental illness.

During my observation of the way the family communicated and shared decisions, I would discretely look for any proof of 'scapegoating', physical or emotional abuse.

Social

I would assess whether the boy's level of social functioning has declined e.g. social withdrawal and whether he was appropriately placed with his family.

---

1 Kraeplin (and some earlier psychiatrists) described a type of schizophrenia in mentally retarded individuals called *pfropfschizophrenie*.

Physical examination

I would conduct a thorough physical and neurological examination. Particular attention would be paid to deficits in hearing or vision.

If multiple or non-accidental fractures are suspected, I would need to arrange a full skeletal (including skull) X-ray.

An electroencephalogram (EEG) would be required if epilepsy is suspected.

Differential diagnosis/diagnostic formulation

The main diagnostic categories are:

(a) Disorders related to the cause of the handicap (e.g. *Down's syndrome, Lesch-Nyhan syndrome*).

(b) A concurrent mental illness (e.g. Affective or psychotic disorder)

(c) An organic disorder (e.g. epilepsy), or

(d) Physical illness e.g. a urinary tract infection producing septicaemia, somatic pain, or worsening sensory deficits.

Frequently, there is no easily diagnosable disorder and the SIB is usually the result of a combination of psychological and social factors e.g. progressive deterioration in function and a decrease in the family's ability to cope with his behaviour.

MANAGEMENT

General opening/special features of the case

The priority would be to try and treat the boy in the community using a multidisciplinary approach. If the SIB was due to a mixture of progressive intellectual deterioration and a decrease in the family's ability to cope with his behaviour the following treatments would be undertaken.

Biological
I would use a dopamine receptor antagonist (e.g. *chlorpromazine*) in the short term to reduce arousal. If pharmacological agents are indicated in the long term, I would consider the addition of *lithium, carbamazepine* or an *opiate receptor antagonist*. The boy would be fitted with a crash helmet for his own protection.

Psychological
With the psychologist, I would set up a behavioural programme using rewards and negative reinforcement (i.e. a *token economy*). All those involved in the boy's care would be familiarised with the programme to ensure that it is consistently applied.

Social

With the social workers, I would make arrangements for the family to be counselled at regular intervals and organise for the family to get practical relief, e.g. child minding, day centre, recreation, holidays or brief hospitalisation. Other members of the multidisciplinary team e.g. the occupational therapists would be asked to help with planning for the boy's future and maximising his skills in as *'normal'* an environment as possible.

REFERENCES AND FURTHER READING

Bicknell J. Living with a mentally handicapped member of the family. *Postgraduate Medical Journal* 1982; 58: 597-605.

Gelder M, Gath D, Mayou R eds. *Oxford Textbook of Psychiatry* (second edition). Oxford: Oxford University Press, 1989: Chapter 21 p 830-51.

Hill P. Behaviour modification with children. *British Journal of Hospital Medicine* January 1982: 51-60.

Oliver C. Self-injurious behaviour in people with a mental handicap. *Current Opinion in Psychiatry* 1988; 1: 567-71.

Wolfensberger W. The definition of normalisation – update, problems, disagreements and misunderstandings. In: Flynn RJ and Nitsch KE. *Normalisation, Social Integration and Community Services*. Baltimore: University Park Press, 1980.

CHAPTER 23

COMPLICATIONS OF PHARMACOTHERAPY

QUESTION 23A

At the depot clinic, you have been asked to see a 50 year old woman who has been receiving neuroleptic medication (fluphenazine 80 mg every fortnight) for the last ten years. She has a diagnosis of chronic schizophrenia, and is often hard to motivate. Additionally, she has neither relapsed nor had any positive symptoms of schizophrenia during that period. On routine examination, however, you notice that her tongue is writhing in her mouth and she is puffing her cheeks.

What is your diagnosis?

Briefly, list your treatment.

ANSWER 23A

See algorithm.

TREATMENT PLAN

My diagnosis would be *tardive dyskinesia* (TD), the central features of which are *orofacial dyskinesia* although the muscles of the limb and trunk could also become involved. The disorder has been associated with D_2 *receptor supersensitivity* due to neuroleptic drugs, and left unchecked, it follows a chronic course; involvement of the respiratory muscles could endanger her life.

Firstly, I would confirm the diagnosis; a neurological examination would be undertaken to exclude other movement disorders such as tardive dystonia, or catatonia (i.e. stereotypies associated with the schizophrenic process itself).

Secondly, although she has several high-risk factors – female sex, middle age, long-term neuroleptic treatment, negative features of schizophrenia – it would be essential to look for others such as an early onset of drug-induced movement disorders, evidence of brain damage or intellectual impairment, and affective symptoms.

Thirdly, because she has been asymptomatic for ten years, provided her background was stable and supportive – *low expressed emotion* (EE) – I would gradually reduce the medication, and

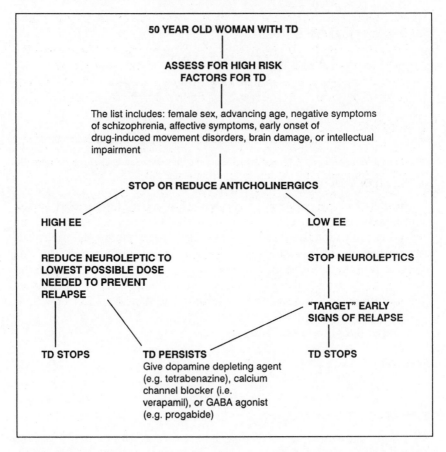

50 YEAR OLD WOMAN WITH TD

**ASSESS FOR HIGH RISK
FACTORS FOR TD**

The list includes: female sex, advancing age, negative symptoms
of schizophrenia, affective symptoms, early onset of
drug-induced movement disorders, brain damage, or intellectual
impairment

STOP OR REDUCE ANTICHOLINERGICS

HIGH EE

LOW EE

**REDUCE NEUROLEPTIC TO
LOWEST POSSIBLE DOSE
NEEDED TO PREVENT
RELAPSE**

STOP NEUROLEPTICS

**"TARGET" EARLY
SIGNS OF RELAPSE**

TD STOPS

TD PERSISTS
Give dopamine depleting agent
(e.g. tetrabenazine), calcium
channel blocker (i.e.
verapamil), or GABA agonist
(e.g. progabide)

TD STOPS

eventually, stop it; any anticholinergic medication would also be
stopped. I would also teach her, and her family, how to recognise the
early signs of a relapse, and stress the importance of maintaining a
low EE environment; treatment would be at "**targetted**" at these
prodromal symptoms using medication with a low liability to produce
TD such as *sulpride or clozapine*.[1]

Fourthly, if she was from a high EE family, the risk of relapse would
be too great to stop the drug; instead, I would carry out a gradual
dose reduction, and aim for the lowest possible dose[2] required for

---

1   Because clozapine has a comparatively high risk of producing agranulocytosis
    (a cumulative annual rate of approximately 2%), regular haematological
    monitoring would be essential. See Kane JM, Honigfield G, Singer J et al.
    Clozapine for the treatment-resistant schizophrenia. *Archives of General Psy-
    chiatry* 1988; 45: 789–96.

2   Low dose neuroleptic treatment would not necessarily reduce the risk of TD;
    social functioning may, however, be improved. "Drug holidays" do not reduce
    the risk of TD.

maintenance. If practicable, I would also consider psychological intervention to reduce EE.

Fifthly, should the TD persist, despite the cessation of neuroleptics, I would treat her with tetrabenazine. Calcium channel blockers (e.g. verapamil or diltiazem), and gamma aminobutyric acid *(GABA) agonists* (e.g. progabide or sodium valproate) would be useful alternatives.

REFERENCES AND FURTHER READING

Barnes TRE. Tardive dyskinesia: risk factors, pathophysiology and treatment. In: *Recent Advances in Clinical Psychiatry Volume 6* (p 185–207), K. Granville-Grossman (editor). London: Churchill Livingstone, 1988.

Barnes TRE, Liddle PF, Curson DA. Negative symptoms, tardive dyskinesia and depression in chronic schizophrenia. *British Journal of Psychiatry* 1989, supplement 7: 99–103.

Gelder M, Gath D, Mayou R. *Oxford Textbook of Psychiatry* (second edition). Oxford: Oxford University Press, 1989; chapter 17 p 647–9.

Jolley AG, Hirsch SR, McRink A et al. Trial of brief neuroleptic prophylaxis for selected outpatients: clinical outcome at one year follow-up. *British Medical Journal* 1989; 298: 985–90.

QUESTION 23B

You have been asked to come urgently to the ward because a 17 year old boy who has been given large intramuscular doses of a high-potency neuroleptic to control his symptoms of mania has become pyrexial (temp 38.5 °C, breathless, tremulous, and "rigid".

Briefly, discuss the diagnosis.

What is the differential diagnosis?

How would you treat this acute situation?

What pharmacological precautions would you take with his aftercare?

ANSWER 23B

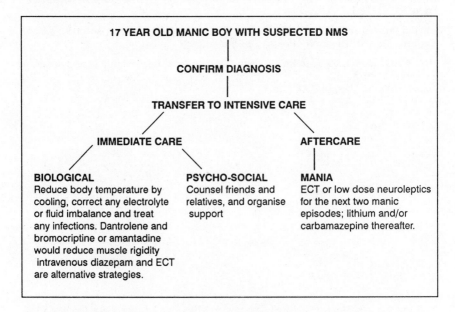

DIAGNOSIS AND DIFFERENTIAL DIAGNOSIS

The most likely diagnosis is *neuroleptic malignant syndrome (NMS)*. Though NMS is commonly associated with schizophrenia, it could also occur in affective disorder. Usually, but not exclusively, *high-potency neuroleptic medication* has been aetiologically linked with its development – suggesting that *central dopamine deficiency*, particularly in the basal ganglia, diencephalon, and anterior hypothalamus could be responsible; often, *catatonic excitement* precedes it, and in some cases, has been hypothesised to cause it.

Other possibilities include: *malignant hyperpyrexia* (MH) – an autosomal dominant condition characterised by an abnormal muscle reaction to anaesthetic agents; *anticholinergic poisoning* (the skin is hot but dry, and there is no tremor or rigidity); *encephalitis*; *heat stroke* (in hot climates); and *lethal catatonia* (very rare nowadays, and described before the advent of neuroleptics).

TREATMENT

General opening/special features of the case

NMS is a medical emergency with a high mortality rate (40%).

Biological
Firstly, I would confirm the diagnosis by conducting a thorough exploration of the nature, onset, and progression of his symptoms – characteristically, there is rapid onset (between 24 and 72 hours) of widespread muscle rigidity with extrapyramidal signs (e.g. cogwheel rigidity), catatonia (rarely), clouding of consciousness (*stupor* or *coma* might supervene), pyrexia and autonomic disturbance (tachycardia, labile blood pressure, profuse sweating and salivation, and urinary incontinence). Elevation of creatinine phosphokinase (CPK), and a leucocytosis would be expected on serological examination.

Secondly, I would stop neuroleptic treatment immediately.

Thirdly, because of the severity of his symptoms, especially the breathing difficulty, it would be safest to arrange his transfer to an intensive care unit.

Fourthly, body cooling would be undertaken to reduce the pyrexia, and any fluid or electrolyte imbalance or infection (pneumonia is common) would be treated. Active treatment of the muscle rigidity, with the combination of *dantrolene* and either *bromocriptine* or *amantadine*, would be more effective than supportive measures. Alternatively, a *slow intravenous* infusion of *diazepam* could also be helpful. As a last resort, particularly if manic symptoms persist, I would give *electroconvulsive therapy* (ECT).

Psycho-social
Fifthly, I would offer supportive counselling to his friends and family.

Dilemmas about aftercare

The early onset and severity of his manic symptoms would suggest a poor prognosis. Though lithium and carbamazepine are effective prophylactic agents which have not been associated with NMS, it would not be appropriate to commence their use on the basis of a single attack of mania. Thus, I would treat the next two episodes of mania with ECT, after which the merits of prophylactic treatment would be reviewed.

Should antidepressants be indicated for the treatment of depression, I would be careful about the choice of tricyclic antidepressant (some tricyclics, for example dothiepin have been linked with NMS),

134 SOLVING CONUNDRUMS IN CLINICAL PSYCHIATRY

and I would avoid the combination of a tricyclic and a monoamine oxidase inhibitor; ECT would be an alternative strategy. Lithium could be used prophylactically.

REFERENCES AND FURTHER READING

Cohen BM, Baldessarini RJ, Pope HG et al. Neuroleptic malignant syndrome. *New England Journal of Medicine* 1985; 313: 1293.

Gelder M, Gath D, Mayou R. *Oxford Textbook of Psychiatry* (second edition). Oxford: Oxford University Press, 1989; chapter 7 p 649–50.

Kellam AMP. The neuroleptic malignant syndrome, so called: a survey of the world literature. *British Journal of Psychiatry* 1987; 150: 752–9.

Mann SC, Carof SN, Bleir HR et al. Lethal catatonia. *American Journal of Psychiatry* 1986; 143: 1374–81.

Perris C. A survey of bipolar and unipolar recurrent depressive psychosis. *Acta Psychiatrica Scandinavica* 1966; supplement 184.

CHAPTER 24
PSYCHOGENIC REGIONAL PAIN

QUESTION 24

You have been asked by a consultant physician to see a 30 year old single woman who has been investigated by him, and several other colleagues for a "second opinion", for a pain in the right side of her face of two years duration, which has not responded to symptomatic treatment with analgesics.

How would you assess her? What is the differential diagnosis? How would you treat the most common presentation?

ANSWER 24

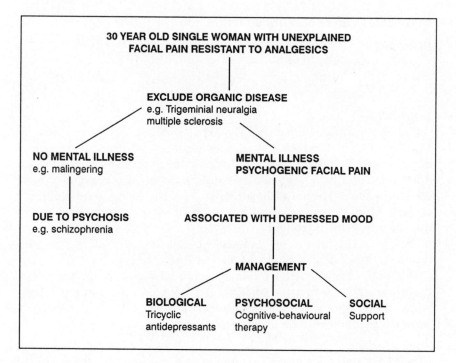

ASSESSMENT

General opening/special features of the case

Because the patient has had several previous consultations with a negative outcome, I would be mindful when I see her that she may be anxious, suspicious, or frankly resentful of doctors; her resentment would be greater if she had been told it was "all in her mind", or if she was convinced that her symptoms were entirely physical in origin. Thus, I would exercise great tact and sensitivity, and assure her that I was taking her symptoms seriously; that is, the diagnosis of a mental disorder would only be made on *positive grounds*, not on the exclusion of physical disorder. I would emphasise that the physician and I were working together as a team on her problems.

Sources of history

I would separately interview the patient and any reliable informants, and review all her medical notes (including those compiled by her general practitioner); a *life chart* would simplify the analysis of this information.

History and mental state examination

Biological

I would look for a family history of either a physical or a mental disorder, and for any proof of *depression, anxiety*, or psychosis.

I would also look for neurological causes.

Psychological

While assessing the onset and progression of her symptoms, I would look specifically for factors which would suggest that the pain was psychogenic. For example, the pain could: be associated with unpleasant *life events*; have a *symbolic significance* (e.g. a parent may have died from a facial tumour); be inconsistent with the neuronal anatomy of the region; be severe enough to prevent sleep, but, paradoxically, not cause early wakening; be unresponsive to all conventional means of amelioration (including analgesics). The reaction of friends and relatives to her disability would also be important.

I would carefully assess her *personality*: focusing on her interpretation and *coping style* towards her pain; interpersonal relationships, her outlook on life and hopes for the future. Evidence of *secondary gain* would be important.

Social

I would evaluate: her level of support in the community; the financial and occupational consequences of her disability; and look for any benefits for maintaining a "sick role".

Physical examination

I would carry out a thorough physical and neurological examination, and review the investigations that have been done. If these findings are unremarkable, I would re-assure the patient, and, firmly but politely, emphasise that this intense level of examination would not be repeated. If new symptoms were to develop, I would not ignore them; a brief re-examination of the patient, limited to the presenting problem, would suffice, unless there is clear evidence of physical disease.

Differential diagnosis

Trigeminal neuralgia, and multiple sclerosis would be important neurological disorders to exclude.

Psychogenic facial pain could be caused by: a reaction to a stressful event; a "masked" emotional disorder such as depression or anxiety; a personality style of exaggeration (i.e. hysterical overlay), preoccupation with disease, or a psychotic illness. She could also be malingering.

MANAGEMENT

The most likely diagnosis is of psychogenic regional pain with depressed mood.

My aim would be to: allay her fears of physical illness; improve her knowledge about the nature of her symptoms; alleviate her pain; and to treat any associated disturbance of mood.

Biological
I would prescribe a tricyclic antidepressant, not only for its antidepressant action, but also for its analgesic properties. I would review her regularly (fortnightly), and set firm limits on the length of her treatment (usually six months) and of each interview.

Psychological
I would provide appropriate, but not blanket reassurance, which could be patronizing, and undermine my relationship with the patient. I would counsel her, pointing out the relationship between her mood and pain. If, however, this is ineffective, I would adopt a cognitive-behavioural approach; other clinicians may opt for interpersonal psychotherapy.

Social
I would encourage her to seek the support of friends and relatives, and to try and maintain as normal a lifestyle as possible.

Differential diagnosis

See algorithm.

REFERENCES AND FURTHER READING

Feinmann C. Psychogenic regional pain. *British Journal of Hospital Medicine* 1990; 43: 123–7.

Gelder M, Gath D, Mayou R. *Oxford Textbook of Psychiatry* (second edition). Oxford: Oxford University Press, 1989; chapter 12 p 412–7.

Sharpe M. The use of graphical life charts in psychiatry. *British Journal of Hospital Medicine* 1990; 44: 44–7.

Smith GR, Monson RA, Ray DC. Psychiatric consultation in somatisation disorder. *New England Journal of Medicine* 1986; 314: 1407–13.

Weatherall DJ, Leddingham JCG, Warrell DA. *Oxford Textbook of Medicine* (second edition). Oxford: Oxford University Press, 1987.

CHAPTER 25

THE IRRITATING PATIENT

QUESTION 25

After five minutes into the interview with a patient, the psychiatrist becomes irritable, and starts to think about "getting rid of the patient".
What are the likely causes?
How could this situation be dealt with?

ANSWER 25

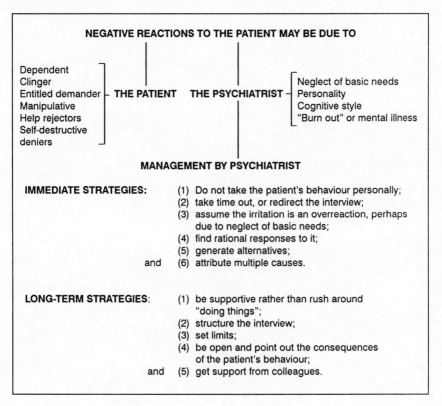

NEGATIVE REACTIONS TO THE PATIENT MAY BE DUE TO

Dependent
Clinger
Entitled demander
Manipulative
Help rejectors
Self-destructive
deniers
— **THE PATIENT** **THE PSYCHIATRIST** —
Neglect of basic needs
Personality
Cognitive style
"Burn out" or mental illness

MANAGEMENT BY PSYCHIATRIST

IMMEDIATE STRATEGIES:
(1) Do not take the patient's behaviour personally;
(2) take time out, or redirect the interview;
(3) assume the irritation is an overreaction, perhaps due to neglect of basic needs;
(4) find rational responses to it;
(5) generate alternatives;
and (6) attribute multiple causes.

LONG-TERM STRATEGIES:
(1) be supportive rather than rush around "doing things";
(2) structure the interview;
(3) set limits;
(4) be open and point out the consequences of the patient's behaviour;
and (5) get support from colleagues.

GENERAL OPENING

Negative reactions such as irritation are common to us all. If, however, they are directed at the patient, it could lead to unprofessional behaviour, and poor clinical judgements and management.

Unless these reactions are examined by the psychiatrist with openness and self-awareness, they could result in a sense of futility, helplessness or of not being appreciated, or *"burn-out"*.

Negative reactions could arise from specific factors in either the patient or the psychiatrist.

FACTORS SPECIFIC TO THE PATIENT

While psychiatrists are not universal in their response to individual patients, *four types of patient* would appear more likely to provoke a negative reaction. These include the: (a) *dependent clinger* – someone who, at first, flatters the doctor (e.g. "only you can help me, you are the best"), but as time goes by, requests almost constant reassurance; usually, there are numerous phone calls, and demands for appointments; (b) *entitled demander* – a well educated patient who claims to "know his rights", and always wants his own way. The manner is usually one of veiled threats and complaints, or there may be repeated requests for a "second opinion" – doctors and lawyers are probably overrepresented in this group; (c) *manipulative help rejector* – these patients are superficially (especially verbally) compliant, but seek to undermine their treatment in other ways. For instance, they may reject important parts of their treatment plan, stop medication, or threaten suicide. The psychiatrist is usually worried that by admitting to the patient that matters are not improving, despite all that is being offered, the relationship between them would deteriorate further; and (d) the *self-destructive denier* – these patients repeatedly harm themselves in some way (e.g. multiple overdosers, alcoholics who fail to stop drinking despite serious medical complications). Frequently, there have been fruitless attempts to engage the patient, who may also have been hostile in treatment; often, there is a common feeling that the patient is refusing, or forcing others to take up his/her responsibilities.

These four types of patient produce negative reactions in the psychiatrist because their need for dependence is overwhelming, and the maladaptive responses of the patient distort the doctor-patient relationship. Interestingly, while some psychiatrists may feel irritated by such patients or develop other negative reactions, others develop a need to "rescue" the patient from themselves.

FACTORS SPECIFIC TO THE PSYCHIATRIST

These fall in to *four broad categories*. They include: (a) *the neglect of the psychiatrist's own basic needs* such as adequate sleep and nourishment; (b) *a personality, self-esteem, or sense of competence* that is easily bruised, demoralised or prejudiced; (c) *cognitive distortions* such as *arbitrary inference* (i.e. rushing to conclusions with insufficient information), *all or nothing thinking* and *personalisation* (taking too much blame for the patient's problems; and (d) *"burn out"*[1] or *overt mental illness* (commonly, depression).

MANAGEMENT

The cause of the irritation (negative reaction) is likely to be multifactorial; "burn out", emotional problems, or overt mental illness would require specific treatments.

Refer to the algorithm for the immediate and long-term management strategies.

REFERENCES AND FURTHER READING

Beck AT. *Cognitive Therapy and Emotional Disorders*. New York: International Universities Press, 1976.

Groves JE. Taking care of the hateful patient. *New England Journal of Medicine* 1978; 298: 883–7.

Mayou R. Burnout. *British Medical Journal* 1987; 295: 284–5.

---

1 *Burnout syndrome* is a condition in which care providers become uninterested and irritable with their patients.

CHAPTER 26

DEMENTIA
AND
PSEUDODEMENTIA

QUESTION 26A

You have been asked to see an elderly couple about whom there is some concern. The wife's daughter says that her mother is covered in bruises and burns, and when she asks about what has caused them, she refuses to discuss the matter further. Despite the general practitioner's request to visit the couple, the husband has refused to see him and also denied access to his wife.

What are the salient points of how you would assess the situation further? What would your management be?

ANSWER 26A

See algorithm.

ASSESSMENT

General opening/special features of the case

This is a difficult case for a number of reasons. It seems likely that the patient's husband is implicated in producing the bruises and burns to his wife's body. Unfortunately, he has refused to see the general practitioner and is likely to refuse to see me. It is, however, clear that the husband needs to be interviewed to clarify what has been happening to his wife. I would approach the problem by contacting the social services who may be able to allocate a social worker with experience in dealing with such situations to this case with whom I would make a joint assessment; also, there may be departmental guidelines[1] for dealing with abuse by carers. The social worker and I

---

1 Social Services departments may have local guidelines for dealing with cases of abuse by carers. It is, however, important to note that in the United Kingdom, unlike the United States of America, their powers to legally enforce the removal of victims of such abuse from their homes to a place of safety are restricted to the provisions of the *1983 Mental Health Act* and Section 47 of the *1948 National Assistance Act* which is seldom used). New legislation is, however,

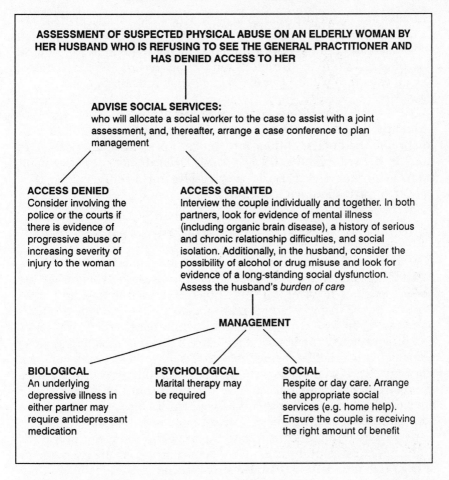

ASSESSMENT OF SUSPECTED PHYSICAL ABUSE ON AN ELDERLY WOMAN BY HER HUSBAND WHO IS REFUSING TO SEE THE GENERAL PRACTITIONER AND HAS DENIED ACCESS TO HER

ADVISE SOCIAL SERVICES:
who will allocate a social worker to the case to assist with a joint assessment, and, thereafter, arrange a case conference to plan management

ACCESS DENIED
Consider involving the police or the courts if there is evidence of progressive abuse or increasing severity of injury to the woman

ACCESS GRANTED
Interview the couple individually and together. In both partners, look for evidence of mental illness (including organic brain disease), a history of serious and chronic relationship difficulties, and social isolation. Additionally, in the husband, consider the possibility of alcohol or drug misuse and look for evidence of a long-standing social dysfunction. Assess the husband's *burden of care*

MANAGEMENT

BIOLOGICAL
An underlying depressive illness in either partner may require antidepressant medication

PSYCHOLOGICAL
Marital therapy may be required

SOCIAL
Respite or day care. Arrange the appropriate social services (e.g. home help). Ensure the couple is receiving the right amount of benefit

would take all practical steps to persuade him to see us including asking someone who knows him or the couple to act as an intermediary. If he refuses to see us, and there is convincing evidence of continuing or increasing severity of abuse towards his wife, it would be necessary (to prevent further injury) to consider, as a last resort, involving the courts and the police to gain access.

Sources of history

We would need to explore relevant details about the couple's relationship and of the patient's injuries from her daughter and any other reliable informants such as friends and relatives, and the general

expected to come into practice in 1993 which will reorganize and co-ordinate the complaints procedure, and the workings of the local authority, social services and the Courts.

practitioner. Particular attention would be paid to any evidence of serious long-standing relationship difficulties (and of physical abuse), social isolation, and social dysfunction in the husband. The general practitioner would be directly asked for any records he may have of her injuries and whether either partner has a history of psychiatric disorder.

At first the couple would be interviewed individually and subsequently, together. Interviewing the couple together would allow us to observe the quality of their interaction: does she irritate or pester him? Is he irritable, hostile, or volatile towards her? Do they communicate effectively? How do they resolve their conflicts? Do they appear to care about each other?

Salient points of the history and mental state examination

The problem with the interview is that at some point we would have to bring up the matter of the patient's injuries. It is unusual for the abused partner to bring up this subject themselves and may even deny it. Thus, using a tactful non-judgemental approach, the husband must, on his own, be asked in detail about the nature, onset and progression of the abuse; often, carers (the husband in this case) respond with relief at being able to discuss their problems with someone else. It would also be important, by making a comprehensive examination of his mental state, to establish that the husband was not suffering from any disorder that would make him prone to violence such as alcohol or drug misuse, depression or dementia.

As well as trying to corroborate the husband's account of events, in the patient's mental state, I would concentrate on the assessment of cognitive function, as I would suspect that she might have some evidence of organic brain disease such as a dementing illness. And I would also want to exclude a mood disorder (especially depression); a possible consequence of the abuse.

A physical examination to identify and treat her injuries, would be carried out.

A full assessment of the *burden of care* borne by the patient's husband would be made. This would include an appraisal of the demands of both a physical (e.g. lifting or coping with incontinence) and emotional (e.g. prolonged periods of sleep disturbance, or a reduced opportunity to socialise or engage in hobbies) nature, and an evaluation of the services (e.g. home help) and benefits[2] they are entitled to.

---

2 A useful book to consult with respect to benefits is the *Disability Rights Handbook* published by the Disability Alliance which is available from the *Alzheimer's Disease Society* head office. The *Alzheimer's Disease Society* at 3rd

MANAGEMENT

General opening/special features of the case

The management plan will be formulated at a multidisciplinary case conference. The safety of the wife is paramount, and therefore, the management hinges on whether it is the patient or her husband that is suffering from a psychiatric disorder or other illness.

Biological

If it seems likely that the patient is suffering from a dementing illness, and it becomes clear that the husband has not been coping and has resorted to violence out of frustration, it might be necessary to arrange a period of *respite or day care* to enable both partners to have a break from each other. This could become a regular feature and might enable both partners to continue to live with each other with a much reduced risk of physical violence. The treatment of a concurrent depressive illness, in addition to appropriate psycho-social measures, could require antidepressant medication.

If alcohol abuse appears to be a particular problem in the husband (by directly contributing towards his aggressive behaviour or accentuating it) help could be sought from a local alcohol advisory service about the best way to manage him. This might include a period of admission for detoxification if he was alcohol dependent.

Psychological

If marital problems are severe, self-referral to *Relate*[3] may be helpful. Regular support throughout the crisis would be helpful, and if I was not able to do this myself I would organise a *Community Nurse* to visit.

Social

If the wife proves to be suffering with a dementing illness and the husband wishes to continue to care for his wife, as well as organising respite care, I would ensure that other agencies involved. And the appropriate services[4] (e.g. *home help* or *meals on wheels*), would be arranged.

A case conference to discuss the implications of the couple's problems and to organise support and monitoring would be essential.

---

floor, Bank Buildings, Fulham Broadway, London SW6 1EP (Telephone: 081-381-31877) can also provide details of a local contact person or carer's group, and publishes a newsletter containing useful practical tips.

3 Relate is a national organization with local branches that provides a counselling service for couples.

4 Advice on how to get in touch with local support groups for *carers* can be obtained from The *National Association for Carers and their Dependents* at 29 Chilworth Mews, London W2 3RG (Telephone: 071-724-7776).

REFERENCES AND FURTHER READING

Homer A C, Gilleard C. Abuse of elderly people by their carers. *British Medical Journal* 1991; 301: 1359–62.

O'Neill O, McCormack P, Walsh JB et al. Elder abuse. *Irish Journal of Medical Science* 1990; 159(2): 48–9.

QUESTION 26B

You have been asked by a general practitioner to make a domicillary visit to see a 70 year old woman. She has been noticed to be crying a lot and seems depressed. Additionally, a neighbour says she has been neglecting herself and when she has tried to help, the woman has become irritable.

What would your management be?

ANSWER 26B

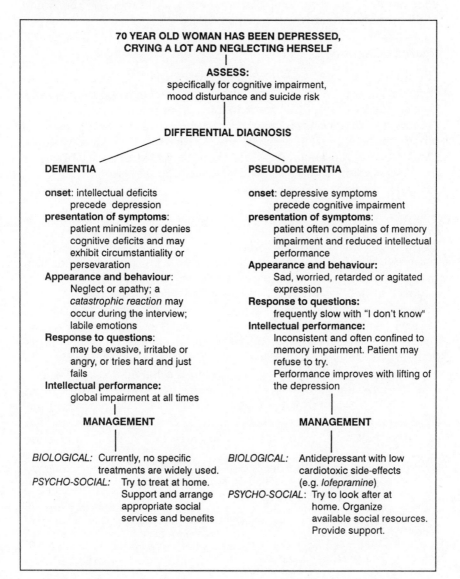

70 YEAR OLD WOMAN HAS BEEN DEPRESSED, CRYING A LOT AND NEGLECTING HERSELF

ASSESS:
specifically for cognitive impairment, mood disturbance and suicide risk

DIFFERENTIAL DIAGNOSIS

DEMENTIA

onset: intellectual deficits precede depression
presentation of symptoms: patient minimizes or denies cognitive deficits and may exhibit circumstantiality or persevaration
Appearance and behaviour: Neglect or apathy; a *catastrophic reaction* may occur during the interview; labile emotions
Response to questions: may be evasive, irritable or angry, or tries hard and just fails
Intellectual performance: global impairment at all times

MANAGEMENT

BIOLOGICAL: Currently, no specific treatments are widely used.
PSYCHO-SOCIAL: Try to treat at home. Support and arrange appropriate social services and benefits

PSEUDODEMENTIA

onset: depressive symptoms precede cognitive impairment
presentation of symptoms: patient often complains of memory impairment and reduced intellectual performance
Appearance and behaviour: Sad, worried, retarded or agitated expression
Response to questions: frequently slow with "I don't know"
Intellectual performance: Inconsistent and often confined to memory impairment. Patient may refuse to try.
Performance improves with lifting of the depression

MANAGEMENT

BIOLOGICAL: Antidepressant with low cardiotoxic side-effects (e.g. *lofepramine*)
PSYCHO-SOCIAL: Try to look after at home. Organize available social resources. Provide support.

ASSESSMENT

General opening/special features of the case

Management would be dependent on assessment.

The main difficulty here is to try and establish what is the underlying cause of her change in behaviour and mood. It is likely to be either an organic disorder such as a dementing process or a functional illness such as depression with an associated cognitive deficit (i.e. *pseudodementia*). It is possible that both disorders could be present at the same time. Assessment should therefore be aimed at differentiating between these two disorders.

Source of history

The important point here is that as far as this assessment is concerned much of the history and observations concerning the patient's mental state would probably come from other informants. As well as obtaining a history from the patient I would also make a point of talking to the spouse (if present), any other relative involved with the patient's care and anyone else, for example a next door neighbour or friend who might be able to shed some light on the problem.

History and mental state examination

Biological

I would obtain as full a history as possible from the patient concerning any change in her mood: when it started and how long it had been going on for. I would also enquire about the patient's sleep, appetite and weight, any past history of depression, and also whether or not there is a family history of depression. I would obtain an alcohol history (if this was possible). I would take a full history of the development of the cognitive impairment and test her cognitive function.[5] Furthermore, I would be mindful that although patients who complain of loss of memory and who tend to highlight their failures may be more likely to be suffering from a depressive disorder than dementia, patients with an early dementia with insight into their condition may also be depressed. I would also make a full assessment of the patient's suicide risk and also carry out a full mental state

---

5 Cognitive function can be formally tested and quantified using the "mini-mental state" examination (see Folstein M F et al. "Mini-mental State". A practical method for grading the cognitive state of patients for the clinician. *Journal of Psychiatric Research* 1975; 12:189–98. Sometimes, patients with dementia may suffer a *catastrophic reaction* (an emotional response to their inability to perform cognitive tasks) and are often evasive or irritable when pressed for answers, and may confabulate. Patients with *pseudodementia* typically respond by saying "I don't know".

examination to exclude the possibility of any other psychiatric disorder such as a psychotic illness.

Psychosocial
From the outset I would wish to empathize with the patient, and attempt to form a good rapport with her.

I would look for any evidence of behavioural disturbance likely to be associated with a dementing disorder such as wandering or aggressive behaviour.

Physical
It might not be appropriate to carry out a physical examination at the first meeting with the patient, especially if no other person is present. I would, therefore, limit my examination to noting any obvious signs of ill-health such as a poor level of hygiene, or neglect, and evidence of gross physical disorder such as anaemia. I would have made general enquiries about the patient's health during the history taking, and this might provide a clue as to a possible cause of her symptoms.

I would arrange with the general practitioner for the patient to have a dementia screen.[6]

MANAGEMENT

General opening/special features of the case

I would attempt to form an opinion about whether the patient could be managed at home. This would depend on: the severity of the disorder and the need for treatment; whether or not the patient is living on her own or has support from a spouse or other relatives; and any associated physical problems that might need treatment. The patient's views should be taken into consideration.

Biological
If the history is suggestive of a dementing process rather than a depressive disorder a decision will need to be taken with the other involved parties (e.g. the general practitioner, Social Worker, District or Community Nurse, and the relatives) as to whether the patient can be managed at home. If there are doubts as to the patient's ability to look after herself or even that she might come to some harm, and increased support can not be arranged in the short term, a period of hospital admission may be indicated. Occasionally admission has to

---

6 A dementia screen is a group of tests and investigations designed to look for a treatable cause. These tests include a full blood count, urea and electrolytes, blood glucose, liver function test, Serum B12, folate, proteins and calcium; syphilis serology, tests of thyroid function, urine culture, skull and chest X ray. The necessity for more specialised tests such as an electroencephalogram and a CT Scan will be dependent on clinical judgement and their availability.

be enforced through the appropriate section of the *1983 Mental Health Act*. On other occasions, and where the patient's own health does not appear to be at risk and where increased support can be organized relatively quickly, it may be preferable to maintain the patient at home in her own surroundings and amongst people she knows. I would stress the importance of good communications between all interested parties so that the patient receives the support she needs.

It may be thought that the patient is more likely to be suffering from a depressive disorder with an associated cognitive defect or behavioural disturbance. Again, a decision has to be taken as to whether she could be managed at home or needs hospital admission. The same criteria apply in that the severity of the illness and the need for treatment as well as the presence or absence of social support would all be important in coming to this decision. A trial of antidepressants would be indicated. I would use a tricyclic antidepressant with low cardiotoxic side-effects (such as *lofepramine*). Clearly, I would want to monitor this process closely, being careful to check that the patient did not suffer with side-effects and was taking her medication correctly.

Sometimes a clear distinction between a diagnosis from an organic and a functional disorder can not be made, and again I would suggest that a trial of antidepressants is indicated. If the patient improves both in mood and in terms of her cognitive performance the diagnosis is more likely to be of a depressive disorder. In contrast, if there is little or no change, dementia would be the favoured option.

Psychosocial
I would look at the possibility of organising increased care for the patient if she remained at home, for example by involving the Social Services Department. I would spend time to inform the patient's relatives of her condition and likely prognosis and put them in touch with support groups such as the *Alzheimer's Disease Society*.[7]

REFERENCES AND FURTHER READING

Differential Diagnosis of Cognitive Impairment from Dementia: an information Bulletin. Washington: Office of Geriatrics and Extended Care, the Letterings Admission, 1985.

---

7 Cross reference Question 26A: *Alzheimer's Disease Society*
The efficacy of specific treatments for Alzheimer's disease such as tetrahydro-aminoacridine and lecithin is currently under investigation. See Summers W K et al. Oral tetrahydroaminoacridine in long-term treatment of senile dementia, Alzheimer's type. *New England Journal of Medicine* 1986; 315: 1241–5 and Chatellier J et al. Tacrine and lecithin in senile dementia of the Alzheimer's type: a multicentre trial. *British Medical Journal* 1990; 300: 495–9.

Gelder M, Gath D, Mayou R. *Oxford Textbook of Psychiatry* (second edition). Oxford: Oxford University Press, 1989; chapter 16 p 610–19.

Lishman W A. *Organic Psychiatry* (second edition). Oxford: Blackwell Scientific Publications, 1989.

CHAPTER 27
ALCOHOLICS AND PROBLEM DRINKERS

QUESTION 27A

You have been asked to see a 30 year old housewife by her general practitioner who says she has been drinking too heavily. Frequently she has been irritable with her husband who has often come home to find her drunk. She has also been neglecting herself and the upkeep of the home.

How would you assess her drinking? What would your management be if she was a problem drinker?

ANSWER 27A

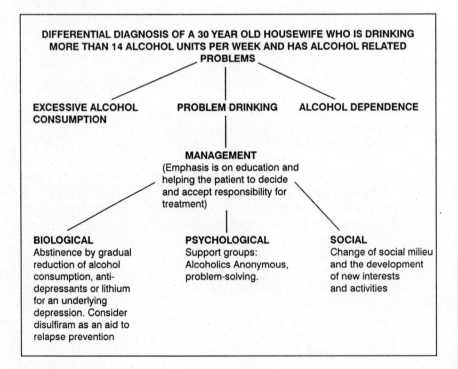

DIFFERENTIAL DIAGNOSIS OF A 30 YEAR OLD HOUSEWIFE WHO IS DRINKING MORE THAN 14 ALCOHOL UNITS PER WEEK AND HAS ALCOHOL RELATED PROBLEMS

EXCESSIVE ALCOHOL CONSUMPTION

PROBLEM DRINKING

ALCOHOL DEPENDENCE

MANAGEMENT
(Emphasis is on education and helping the patient to decide and accept responsibility for treatment)

BIOLOGICAL
Abstinence by gradual reduction of alcohol consumption, anti-depressants or lithium for an underlying depression. Consider disulfiram as an aid to relapse prevention

PSYCHOLOGICAL
Support groups:
Alcoholics Anonymous, problem-solving.

SOCIAL
Change of social milieu and the development of new interests and activities

ASSESSMENT

General opening/special features of the case

I would need to take a full alcohol history as part of the general history and mental state examination.

In this case, three factors could complicate the *alcohol history*. The patient could have concealed her drinking for some time and, there-fore, her husband could harbour feelings of anger or resentment towards her; the patient and her husband could have chosen to ignore her drinking to save embarrassment; and, her husband could also have been misusing alcohol. Thus, it would be important to develop a *therapeutic alliance* that encouraged the lowering of the couples defences, to understand the patient as a woman in her own right, and to provide them with empathetic but accurate feedback.

The aim of my assessment would, therefore, be to determine the severity of drinking by the patient and her husband.

The alcohol history would determine whether she was an *excessive drinker*, a *problem drinker*, or *dependent on alcohol*.

Sources of history

I would interview the patient, ask the general practitioner for further details and, on his own, interview her husband, not only about her drinking pattern, but about his own.

History and mental state examination

An *alcohol history* has seven essential parts.

I would: *firstly*, want to know what her main *problems were*, and their consequences and maintaining factors;

secondly, determine the *onset, nature and progression of the drinking behaviour* – how did drinking start and was it accompanied by any social or peer pressure? When was the first episode of: drinking spirits; drinking regularly or in bouts? How much does she and her husband drink now or spend on alcohol (*excessive alcohol consumption* constitutes >14 and 21 alcohol units/week for women and men respectively)? Where and with whom do they drink?

thirdly, look for evidence of *problem drinking*[1] – has there been any guilt, accusations of excessive drinking or a request to cut down the amount? Was an "*eye opener*" required to withdrawal symptoms in the morning?

The last four questions are known as the "*Cage*" questionnaire – and identify the *stage of change*[2] which has been achieved. Further-

---

1 More than two positive answers on the Cage questionnaire would suggest problem drinking.

more, I would look for *medical consequences* of drinking. For examples, ulcers, liver damage, or neuropsychiatric complications such as blackouts, withdrawal fits, or cognitive impairment (women have a relatively greater risk of alcohol induced physical damage than men because a smaller percentage of their body weight is water);

fourthly, if he/she was a problem drinker, look for evidence of *dependence*. These include a compulsion to drink, salience of drinking, repeated withdrawal symptoms, drinking to avoid withdrawal symptoms, reinstatement of drinking following a period of abstinence, and pharmacological tolerance;

fifthly, assess the *impact of her drinking on her life*; was the marriage stable? Were there any longstanding conflicts, episodes of aggression or sexual difficulties? Were there any financial or legal problems (including drink related motoring offences)?

sixthly, look for evidence of any *other addictive behaviours* including the misuse of other drugs. If there was associated drug misuse, I would be interested in its type, frequency and method of usage (particularly of injectable drugs), any periods of abstinence, and attempts at treatment;

seventhly, look for proof of *psychiatric vulnerability to alcoholism* (by virtue of a family history of alcoholism or depressive spectrum disorder[3]), *a concomitant psychiatric illness* such as depression, anxiety, or a phobic state which could have been precipitated or aggravated by the excessive drinking, and assess *early development*, *personality* and *psycho-social adjustment* (e.g. were there any problems at school such as school refusal or truancy? What were the parents' attitudes to drinking? Were there any longstanding adjustment difficulties such as interpersonal or sexual difficulties? What was the premorbid personality like?).

Physical examination

I would carry out a thorough medical and neurological examination (specifically to look for *liver or neurological complications*), and perform a full blood count and liver function test (to look for a rise in *mean corpuscular volume* and *gamma glutamyltranspeptidase* respectively).

---

2 "The stages of change" include *precontemplation* (no recognition of the need for a change in behaviour), *contemplation* (some recognition but no action), *action* and *maintenance*. See Prochaska J A et al., 1986.

3 Cross reference 27B for depressive spectrum disorder.

MANAGEMENT

General opening/special features of the case

Assuming she was a *problem drinker* I would *educate* her about the risks of excessive alcohol consumption and help her to decide and take responsibility for what to do about it. If she was willing to accept help, her goals should include *abstinence*[4] (at least initially) *relapse prevention*, and *resolving interpersonal social and legal difficulties*. The commonest technique for achieving abstinence is a gradual reduction in alcohol consumption which can be monitored using an *alcohol diary*.

Biological

Because alcohol misuse could itself produce psychological symptoms such as anxiety or depression, it would be prudent to withhold pharmacological treatment for these disorders unless they persist longer than three weeks following abstinence or to have preceded and presumably triggered the excessive drinking. *Antidepressants* or *lithium therapy* could be helpful in treating depressive disorders. I would discuss with the patient the risks and appropriateness of prescribing an *alcohol-sensitizing*[5] *drug* such as *disulfiram* ('Antabuse') as an aid to relapse prevention.

---

4 Clinicians (including examiners) can have strong views about whether or not *controlled drinking* is a more realistic goal than *abstinence* in problem drinkers. In my experience, however, most clinicians would agree that a period of abstinence is desirable even if the long term management plan is controlled drinking. For a review see Chick J, *British Journal of Hospital Medicine* (October) 1986: 241.

5 The use of *alcohol-sensitizing* such as *disulfiram* ('*Antabuse*') as an aid to relapse prevention (particularly in impulsive drinkers) has strong proponents and detractors. It works by inhibiting *alcohol dehydrogenase* in the liver with the consequence that there is an accumulation of acetaldehyde (which causes histamine release) whenever is ingested. This produces flushing (mainly in the face and upper trunk), nausea, vomiting, dizziness and headaches. More serious side effects may occur particularly if large amounts of alcohol are ingested. These include: peripheral neuropathy, impotence, tachycardia, cardiac arrhythmias and cardiovascular collapse (rare) and acute confusional states. Thus, the implied threat of this reaction (often termed a "vicarious conditioned aversive response") acts as a chemical fence for 24 hours after each tablet. Obviously it would be dangerous to prescribe this drug to a patient who intends to continue drinking.
In the last ten years, several controlled trials have investigated the efficacy of disulfiram. The current literature suggests that unless its administration is supervised (e.g. by a spouse or work colleague) as part of the treatment contract and combined with counselling the results are poor. It appears, however, that the longer disulfiram is taken the less likely it is for the patient to return to drinking. This has lead to the suggestion that the drug may reduce the motivation to drink through its effects on biogenic amines; perhaps, principally, by the central inhibition of dopamine beta hydroxylase. Of course, the

Psychological
Self-help would be emphasized. And, I would, therefore, advise her to attend an alcohol support group, such as *Alcoholics Anonymous* to prevent relapse; her husband would be offered the opportunity to attend a family support group (e.g. *Al-Anon*). They could also require marital therapy.

Social
I would adopt a *problem-solving* approach to her remaining difficulties, and reinforce the *educational* message by providing her with a self-help booklet[6]. I would also suggest that she *change her social milieu* to get away from her "drinking" friends and seek stimulating new activities and interests.

Legal difficulties would be dealt with in the appropriate way.

REFERENCES AND FURTHER READING

Camberwell Council of Alcoholism. *Women and Alcohol*. London: Tavistock, 1980.

Edwards G. *The Treatment of Drinking Problems*. London: Grant McIntyre Medical and Scientific Publications, 1982.

Gelder M, Gath D, Mayou R. *Oxford Textbook of Psychiatry* (second edition). Oxford: Oxford University Press 1989; chapter 14 p 514 and 522–37.

Mayfield D, Millard G, Hall P. The CAGE questionnaire: validation of a new alcoholism screening instrument. *American Journal of Psychiatry* 1974; 131: 1121–3.

Prochaska JO, Diclemente CC. Towards a comprehensive model of change. In: Miller W, Heather N (editors). *Treating Addictive Behaviours: Processes of Change*. New York: Plenum, 1986.

Royal College of Psychiatrists. *Alcohol: Our Favourite Drug*. London: Tavistock, 1986.

---

regular taking of the tablet reminds the patient of his problem and can also be a symbolic representation of the supportive role played by the therapist. For reviews see: Sinclair JD, the feasibility of effective psychopharmacological treatments for alcoholism, *British Journal of Addiction* 1987; 82: 1213–23 and Brewer C, Supervised disulfiram in alcoholism, *British Journal of Hospital Medicine*; 35: 116–9.

6 A useful self-help booklet is called *That's the Limit: a Guide to Sensible Drinking* published by the Health Education Authority 1989.

QUESTION 27B

You have been to see a 50 year old married chef on the orthopaedic ward who was brought in to hospital two days ago on account of a fractured femur, for which he has had emergency surgery. He is described as becoming "suddenly aggressive, restless, talking to himself, confused, anxious and tremulous;". How would you assess him and reach a differential diagnosis? If you decide delirium tremens is the most likely diagnosis, how would you manage it?

ANSWER 27B

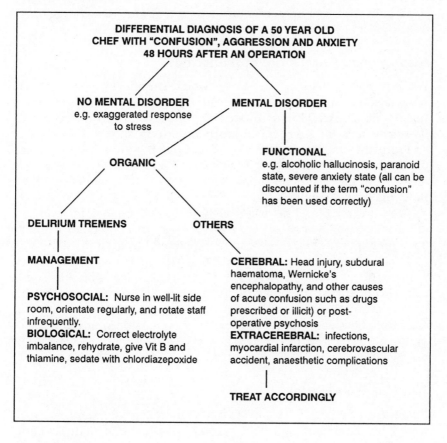

DIFFERENTIAL DIAGNOSIS OF A 50 YEAR OLD CHEF WITH "CONFUSION", AGGRESSION AND ANXIETY 48 HOURS AFTER AN OPERATION

NO MENTAL DISORDER
e.g. exaggerated response to stress

MENTAL DISORDER

ORGANIC

FUNCTIONAL
e.g. alcoholic hallucinosis, paranoid state, severe anxiety state (all can be discounted if the term "confusion" has been used correctly)

DELIRIUM TREMENS

OTHERS

MANAGEMENT

PSYCHOSOCIAL: Nurse in well-lit side room, orientate regularly, and rotate staff infrequently.
BIOLOGICAL: Correct electrolyte imbalance, rehydrate, give Vit B and thiamine, sedate with chlordiazepoxide

CEREBRAL: Head injury, subdural haematoma, Wernicke's encephalopathy, and other causes of acute confusion such as drugs prescribed or illicit) or post-operative psychosis
EXTRACEREBRAL: infections, myocardial infarction, cerebrovascular accident, anaesthetic complications

TREAT ACCORDINGLY

ASSESSMENT

General opening/special features of the case

Management is dependent on assessment.

Although the patient's symptoms are suggestive of an alcohol withdrawal syndrome, it would be prudent to exclude other relevant organic or functional disorders. There is, of course, also the possibility that his symptoms have not been produced by mental disorder.

Since getting a detailed history from such an ill patient is unlikely to be practicable, I would carefully explore other sources of information.

Sources of information

I would seek access to all his medical notes, and if applicable, his psychiatric notes, and telephone his general practitioner for further details.

I would see the patient, and interview his wife and the charge nurse on the ward.

History and mental state examination

While reviewing his medical notes, I would specifically look for conditions associated with excessive alcohol intake, and for a past family history of mental illness (especially of *alcohol dependence* or *depressive spectrum disorder*,[7] or *paranoid disorder*).

From the charge nurse, I would find out if he has had any sleep difficulties (e.g. insomnia, or nightmares), and ensure that the term "confusion" had been used in its proper context (i.e. disorientation for time, place or person).

From his own, and his wife's testimony, I would look for evidence of *alcohol dependence*[8], epilepsy (which may be associated with the fall causing the broken leg), and unexplained blackouts.

In his mental state, I would be particularly interested in the content of his hallucinations (especially if they harbour ideas about harming himself or others). During this acute episode, I would examine his cognitive function for evidence of an *acute organic mental disorder*; after this, however, I would establish if there has been any chronic or progressive memory impairment (i.e. *alcoholic dementia or Korsakoff's psychosis*).

Physical examination

I would undertake a full physical and neurological examination. It would be important to look for common causes of acute organic disturbance such as drugs (prescribed or illicit), post-operative psy-

---

7 For a description of depressive spectrum disorder see Winokur G, *Archives of General Psychiatry* 1971; 24: 135–44.

8 The main features of alcohol dependence are increased salience of drinking; the presence of withdrawal symptoms on repeated occasions, the reinstatement of a dependent drinking pattern following a period of abstinence; and changes in pharmacological tolerance.

chosis, infections (pneumonia or urinary tract infection), head injury with cerebral lacerations or a subdural haematoma, myocardial infarction, or a cerebrovascular accident. And, I would look for specific medical complications of alcohol misuse: jaundice, liver palms, spider naevi and hepatomegaly (i.e. for evidence of *liver involvement*), ocular palsies or nystagmus (which would distinguish *delirium tremens* from *Wernicke's encephalopathy*[9], and for peripheral neuropathy or myopathy. The following investigations would, therefore, be necessary: a full blood count and a liver function test (alcoholics often have a raised *mean corpuscular volume* and *gamma glutamyl transpeptidase* respectively); urea and electrolytes; urine culture and glucose; a chest and skull X-ray.

Differential diagnosis

See algorithm.

MANAGEMENT

General opening/special features of the case

I would treat delirium tremens as a medical emergency; it has an appreciable mortality rate (5%).

Psychosocial
I would nurse him in a brightly lit side-room, orientate him regularly, and keep the rotation of staff looking after him to a minimum.

Biological
I would ensure that his vital signs (pulse, blood pressure and temperature) were monitored at half hourly intervals (more frequently if necessary).

I would correct any electrolyte imbalance and rehydrate. If he was hypoglycaemic, I would administer *B vitamins* (parentrovite I and II) and *thiamine* (200 mg/day) *before giving glucose* (otherwise, Wernicke's encephalopathy may be precipitated). Infrequently, *ketoacidosis* may be a complication; for this, I would give insulin.

I would give a sedative minor tranquilliser[10] to reduce agitation, ensure rest and sleep, to prevent exhaustion, and to facilitate nursing care; a reducing schedule (over seven days) of *chlordiazepoxide* (starting dose 50–100 mg four times a day), would preferably, be given parenterally.

---

9 Wernicke's encephalopathy is characterised by clouding of consciousness, lateral ophthalmoplegia and nystagmus, ataxia, and peripheral neuropathy.
10 Other tranquillisers which have been used in alcohol withdrawal include chlormethiazole, chlorpromazine or haloperidol (neuroleptics), and paraldehyde.

I would institute prophylactic short-term anticonvulsant therapy, *carbamazepine* or *sodium valproate* at a therapeutic dose level, if there is a significant risk of epilepsy (i.e. by virtue of a family or personal history); intravenous *diazepam* could be substituted for chlordiazepoxide to control convulsions.

REFERENCES AND FURTHER READING

Gelder M, Gath D, Mayou R. *Oxford Textbook of Psychiatry* (second edition). Oxford: Oxford University Press 1989: Chapter 14 p 532–3.

Cutting J. Physical illness and psychosis. *British Journal of Psychiatry* 1980; 136: 109–19.

Cutting J. Neuropsychiatric complications of alcoholism. *British Journal of Hospital Medicine* (April 1982): 335–42.

Gillanpaa ML. Treatment of alcohol withdrawal symptoms. *British Journal of Hospital Medicine* (April 1982): 343–50.

Jarman CMB and Kellett JM. 1979. *Alcoholism in the General Hospital* 2 469–71.

CHAPTER 28

DYNAMIC PSYCHOTHERAPY: ASSESSMENT FOR TREATMENT

QUESTION 28

You have been asked to take on a 23 year old secretary for dynamic psychotherapy who has been feeling low for 3 years. She has had several boyfriends in the last year because feels she always needs someone around. She does not have a depressive illness.

How would you assess her?

ANSWER 28

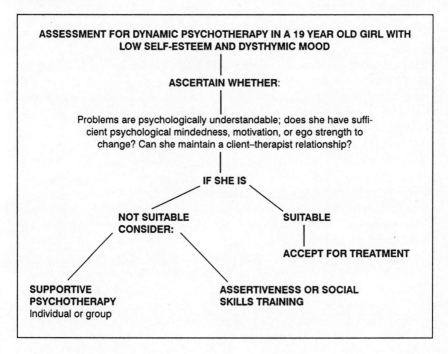

ASSESSMENT FOR DYNAMIC PSYCHOTHERAPY IN A 19 YEAR OLD GIRL WITH LOW SELF-ESTEEM AND DYSTHYMIC MOOD

ASCERTAIN WHETHER:

Problems are psychologically understandable; does she have sufficient psychological mindedness, motivation, or ego strength to change? Can she maintain a client–therapist relationship?

IF SHE IS

NOT SUITABLE CONSIDER:

SUITABLE

ACCEPT FOR TREATMENT

SUPPORTIVE PSYCHOTHERAPY
Individual or group

ASSERTIVENESS OR SOCIAL SKILLS TRAINING

ASSESSMENT

General opening/special features of the case

The problems of low self-esteem, dysthymic mood and interpersonal problems could, theoretically, be helped by *dynamic psychotherapy*; the aim of my assessment, however, would be to find out if she herself was suitable, and if not, to ascertain what other kind of therapy she could benefit from. And we would both need to decide whether we could work together as client and therapist.

Though this would be her initial interview with me, she would, in all probability, have previously seen up to two other doctors, (including a psychiatrist); thus, she could be irritated or resentful at having been "passed on" yet again. I would acknowledge these feelings, should they arise, and emphasise the need to *take my own history*. Additionally, she could be uncertain about what to expect in psychotherapy, and apprehensive about having to confide in a stranger. I would educate her about what to expect in psychotherapy and suggest that she read a suitable "lay man's" guide[1]

Source of history

An interview with the patient.

History
Firstly, I would ascertain if her problems could be understood in psychological terms, and whether she had the *psychological minded-ness* to see them in this way? *Hypothesis testing* would be used: For example, "could your need to be in a relationship, no matter how unsatisfactory, be related to your low opinion of yourself?"

Secondly, I would assess her *motivation* to change.

Thirdly, if she was motivated to change, I would determine whether she had the capacity to do so. This would depend on whether she had sufficient *ego strength* – the ability to bear the inner tensions that would arise from confronting conflicts without decompensating and to give up maladaptive patterns of behaviour such as remaining in an obviously destructive relationship.

Fourthly, I would find out if she would be able to maintain a client-therapist relationship. This would include practical considerations such as turning up regularly and on time for her appointments, and ability to maintain ego boundaries; that is, between sessions she should be capable of functioning as a responsible adult without, habitually, "*acting out*[2], or becoming dependent on the

---

1 Examples of useful general information books are : Quillian S. *The Counselling Handbook*. Northamptonshire: Thorsons (1990), and L Knight. *Talking to a Stranger*. Glasgow: Fontana, (1986).

therapy. Thus, evidence of poor impulse control, excessive depend-ence, borderline personality, or a history of psychosis would be contraindications to dynamic psychotherapy.

Should she not be suitable for dynamic psychotherapy, I would consider whether she would benefit from supportive therapy (individ-ual or group) or assertiveness training or social skills. She could also benefit from reading a practical self-help book[3]

REFERENCES AND FURTHER READING

Gelder M, Gath D, Mayou R. *Oxford Textbook of Psychiatry* (second edition). Oxford: Oxford University Press, 1989; chapter 18 p 694–723.

Malan D. *The Frontier of Brief Psychotherapy*. New York: Plenum, 1977

Sandler J, Dare C, Holder A. *The Patient and the Analyst*: the basis of the psychoanalytic process. London: Allen and Unwin, 1973.

Storr, A. *The Art of Psychotherapy*. Oxford: Heinemann Medical Books, 1979.

---

2 Acting out" is the direct expression of an unconscious wish to impulse in action to avoid being conscious of the accompanying effect. The unconscious fantasy, involving objects, is lived out impulsively in behaviour, thus gratifying the impulse more than prohibiting against it. On a chronic level, acting out involves giving into impulses to avoid the tension that would result from postponement of expression. From: Kaplan HI, Sadock BJ. *Synopsis of Psychiatry* (fifth edition). Baltimore: Williams and Wilkins, 1988.

3 Recommended self-help books include: Burns DD. *Feeling Good*. New York: William Morrow and Company Inc. (1980), and, Lindefield G. *Assert Yourself*. Northamptonshire: Thorsons, (1986).

CHAPTER 29

ETHICS AND GENETIC COUNSELLING: HUNTINGTON'S CHOREA

QUESTION 29

A 20 year old married woman has been sent to see you for advice because she wishes to have a family. Her husband's father died in his 30's of a movement disorder characterised by unintentional jerks, as did his grandfather. Her husband is the same age as her, and asymptomatic.

What disorder do you suspect her husband could be a carrier of?
What would your advice be?

ANSWER 29

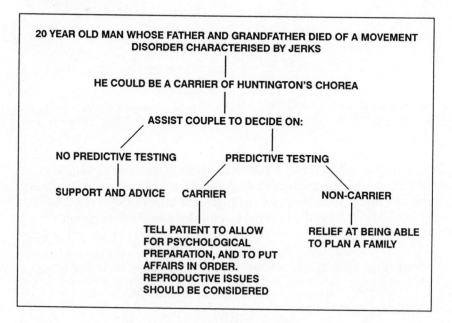

20 YEAR OLD MAN WHOSE FATHER AND GRANDFATHER DIED OF A MOVEMENT DISORDER CHARACTERISED BY JERKS
|
HE COULD BE A CARRIER OF HUNTINGTON'S CHOREA
|
ASSIST COUPLE TO DECIDE ON:

NO PREDICTIVE TESTING   PREDICTIVE TESTING

SUPPORT AND ADVICE   CARRIER   NON-CARRIER

TELL PATIENT TO ALLOW   RELIEF AT BEING ABLE
FOR PSYCHOLOGICAL   TO PLAN A FAMILY
PREPARATION, AND TO PUT
AFFAIRS IN ORDER.
REPRODUCTIVE ISSUES
SHOULD BE CONSIDERED

DIAGNOSIS

He could be a carrier of *Huntington's Chorea* (HC), an autosomal dominant, and ultimately fatal condition characterised by progressive choreic movements which are often accompanied by mental changes (e.g. *paranoid psychosis, dementia, depression* and *suicide* are common). It is due to selective loss of gamma aminobutyric acid *(GABA) neurones* in the *basal ganglia* (especially the caudate and putamen) and *cortex*; additionally, *dopamine hypersensitivity* is produced by impairment of GABA and glutamic acid decarboxylase (GAD) activity.

Early onset HC may be predominantly transmitted from father to son, and the disorder occurs, comparatively, about ten years earlier in the children of affected males than females.

ADVICE

The couple require *genetic counselling* which could be undertaken by a psychiatrist or a trained counsellor and a geneticist. An *educational approach* in counselling, the transfer of essential information by packing it into personally meaningful units, would be used to help them reach a decision about their dilemma: should they choose to exercise their right to know by *predictive testing* (using a polymorphic DNA marker, G8) or try to live with the uncertainty of not knowing. Should he, however, develop the disease, the *burden of care* would rest with his wife, and if she fell pregnant, there would be a 50% chance of having an affected foetus (and a decision would have to be made about whether or not she should continue with the pregnancy). Although predictive testing would, strictly, only require the informed consent of the husband, it would be crucial to explore his wife's feelings about it and to specifically assess the potential impact of a positive or negative test result on the marriage. Furthermore, predictive testing raises three other important ethical questions: the possibility of inaccurate predictions from the test – because there is at present a 5% risk of error, a positive carrier status result should not be taken as a pre-symptomatic diagnosis (it could be argued that this small amount of uncertainty gives high-risk individuals a reasonable degree of hope); identified carriers could be unable to cope with the burden of knowledge – mental illness, or suicide could result; and the test could be misused – for example, insurance companies could refuse to cover people at high-risk of being carriers if they refuse testing. Usually, confirmation of non-carrier status would be a relief.

Regardless of whether the couple decide on testing, they would need *supportive counselling* which could be provided by a local branch of the HC support group[1]

In my opinion, should the couple decide on testing, I would be honest about the result because it would afford them the opportunity to prepare themselves psychologically, and to put their affairs in order; interestingly, high-risk carrier status does not always deter reproductive intention, or reduce sexual activity.

At risk individuals should be entered on a *genetic register*.

REFERENCES AND FURTHER READING

Anonymous. On telling dying patients the truth (editorial). *Journal of Medical Ethics* 1982; 8: 115–6.

Bolt JMW. Huntington's Chorea in the West of Scotland. *British Journal of Psychiatry* 1970; 116: 259–70.

Crawford DIO, Harris R. Ethics of predictive testing for Huntington's Chorea: the need for more information. *British Medical Journal* 1986; 293: 249–51.

Gelder M, Gath D, Mayou R. *Oxford Textbook of Psychiatry* (second edition). Oxford: Oxford University Press, 1989; chapter 11 p 366–8.

Gusella JF, Wexler NS, Conneally PM et al. A polymorphic DNA marker genetically linked to Huntington's disease. *Nature* 1983; 306: 234–8.

Seymour K. Psychological aspects of genetic counselling: A critical review of the literature dealing with education and reproduction. *American Journal of Medical Genetics* 1989; 34: 340–53.

---

1 The *Association to Combat Huntington's Chorea*. Two useful general information booklets include *Huntington's Chorea: A Booklet for the Family Doctors of Patients with the Disease* published by the Committee on Huntington's Chorea of the Central Council for the Disabled and the National Fund for Research in to Crippling Diseases, and *on Nursing Huntington's Chorea*, Gardham F (editor), published by the *Association to Combat Huntington's Chorea* (1982)..

CHAPTER 30

THE MENTALLY ABNORMAL OFFENDER AND THE MENTAL HEALTH ACT

QUESTION 30A

You have been asked to assess, for the purpose of a court report, a 45 year old married woman who has recently been charged with shoplifting. How would you carry this out? What is the differential diagnosis? What advice would you give the court?

ANSWER 30A

See algorithm.

ASSESSMENT

General opening/special features of the case

The purpose of the assessment would be to determine whether she had a mental disorder and to make recommendations to the court about the appropriateness of psychological management.

Sources of history

I would need to interview the patient and her husband (separately at first, and then together) and a reliable informant such as a close relative or friend. A sensitive and non-judgemental approach would be essential.

History and mental state examination

Biological
I would be interested in a family or personal history of mental disorder (particularly *depression* and including phobic anxiety, alcohol or drug misuse, affective psychosis, or schizophrenia) and complaints of recent or chronic physical illness.

167

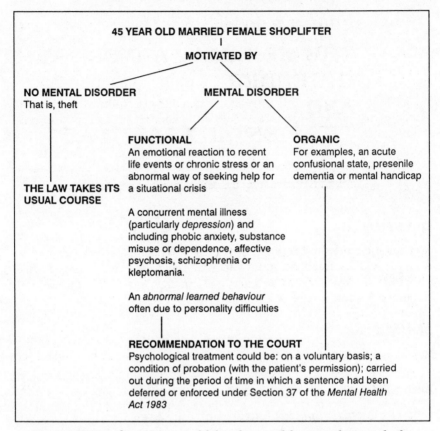

Her cognitive function would be thoroughly tested to exclude an organic condition such as a confusional state, presenile dementia or mental handicap.

Psychological
I would obtain a detailed account of the circumstances surrounding the alleged shoplifting: was it planned? Was there a financial[1] motive? What was her mental state (if determinable) at the time? Did she feel compelled[2] to steal? What was her reaction[3] when she was caught?

---

1 Shoplifting could be a way of raising money to buy alcohol or drugs, or to pay off debts; other methods include prostitution.
2 *Kleptomania*, a compulsion to steal characterized by increasing tension before and relief afterwards is included in the third edition of the *Diagnostic and Statistical Manual of Mental Disorders* (DSM III-R). Washington DC: American Psychiatric Association, 1987.
3 People who shoplift to, inappropriately, draw attention to their emotional distress sometimes experience a temporary sense of relief when they are caught; on the other hand, depressed shoplifters often interpret the humiliation of being caught as deserving punishment for past misdemeanours.

Did she have any previous convictions? Has she shoplifted in the past and how did she feel then? And I would specifically look for evidence of *recent life events* (e.g. bereavement) or *chronic stress* (especially *marital problems*). The shoplifting could either be a direct response to emotional difficulties or an abnormal way of seeking help for them.

I would assess her *personality*. Particular attention would be paid to evidence of poor impulse control, violence or other antisocial behaviours.

Social
A tactful inquiry into her social circumstances and an exploration of her habits and life-style would be essential.

Differential diagnosis
See algorithm

ADVICE TO THE COURT

In English law, shoplifting is dealt with under the *Theft Act 1968*.

The court report should include the history, diagnosis, assessment of the alleged shoplifter's mental state at the time of the offence (if determinable), conclusions and recommendations to the court.

The recommendations must comment on her fitness to plead[4], the appropriateness of treatment, prognosis, and the risk of re-offending. Recommendations prior to the trial could be made for remand in custody for psychiatric reports, remand to a psychiatric hospital for treatment, or transfer from prison to hospital. During the trial, if the alleged shoplifter was found guilty and had a treatable mental disorder, the court could be asked to consider: voluntary treatment, treatment as a condition of probation (the offender must agree to this), deferral of the sentence to allow treatment to take place, or compulsory treatment under Section 37 of the *Mental Health Act 1983*.

REFERENCE AND FURTHER READING

Fisher C. Psychiatric aspects of shoplifting. *British Journal of Hospital Medicine* (March) 1984: 209–12.

Gelder M, Gath D, Mayou R. *Oxford Textbook of Psychiatry* (second edition). Oxford University Press, 1989; Chapter 22 p 886–8.

---

4 A person who is *fit to plead* must understand the nature of the charge, know the difference between pleading guilty and not guilty, and be able to instruct counsel, challenge jurors and follow the evidence presented in court.
   Although there has been much speculation and debate about a specific association between shoplifting and premenstrual tension and the menopause, the evidence, however, remains unconvincing (for a discussion see Gibbens 1971 and Fisher 1984). However, premenstrual tension has, in recent trials, been successfully used to plead mitigation by virtue of psychological disturbance.

Gibbens TCN, Palmer C, Prince J. Mental health aspects of shoplifting. *British Journal of Hospital Medicine* 1971; 3: 612–5.

Gudjonsson GH. Causes of compulsive shoplifting. *British Journal of Hospital Medicine* (September) 1988; 40: 169.

QUESTION 30B

You have on your ward a 19 year old girl with a diagnosis of anorexia nervosa who is 40% below her expected body weight, and is losing more than 2 kg of weight per week. She has now stopped eating and drinking completely because she is "too fat", and she is accusing the staff of wanting her to gain weight too quickly. She says she is discharging herself, and is making for the door.

Would you take any measures to stop her from leaving, if so what?

ANSWER 30B

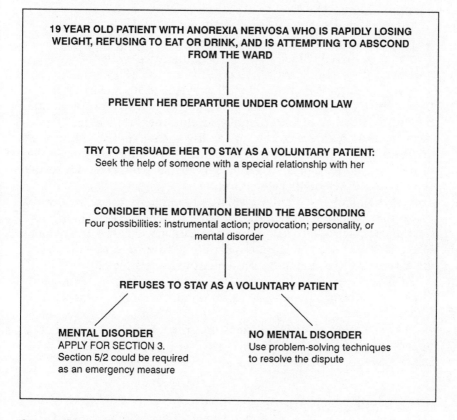

19 YEAR OLD PATIENT WITH ANOREXIA NERVOSA WHO IS RAPIDLY LOSING WEIGHT, REFUSING TO EAT OR DRINK, AND IS ATTEMPTING TO ABSCOND FROM THE WARD

PREVENT HER DEPARTURE UNDER COMMON LAW

TRY TO PERSUADE HER TO STAY AS A VOLUNTARY PATIENT:
Seek the help of someone with a special relationship with her

CONSIDER THE MOTIVATION BEHIND THE ABSCONDING
Four possibilities: instrumental action; provocation; personality, or mental disorder

REFUSES TO STAY AS A VOLUNTARY PATIENT

MENTAL DISORDER
APPLY FOR SECTION 3.
Section 5/2 could be required as an emergency measure

NO MENTAL DISORDER
Use problem-solving techniques to resolve the dispute

General opening/special features of the case

This anorexic girl's life is in danger because of her very low weight, the rapid loss of weight, and her refusal to eat or drink; she, therefore, needs to remain in hospital for treatment.

PLAN TO STOP HER FROM LEAVING

I would: firstly, prevent her from leaving the ward using my powers under common law[5].

Secondly, seek to persuade her to stay as a voluntary patient – the help of a member of staff (or relative if available) with whom she has a special relationship would be sought to negotiate with her – assurances would have to be made that her stay on the ward was in her best interests, her behaviour would not be punished, and that any difficulties she had with the treatment regime would be openly discussed and a written contract drawn up with her before proceeding with a new plan.

Thirdly, consider the four possible reasons for her behaviour – instrumental action (to protest at an excessively stringent programme), personality factors ("testing boundaries" could be part of an antisocial personality, or there could be evidence of secondary gain such as playing one member of staff against the other especially if the treatment plan was inconsistently applied), provocation by another patient or member of staff (usually around meal times), and mental disorder (which could be due to the increasing severity of anorexia nervosa) or the development of new symptoms such as a depressive or psychotic illness, or an organic disturbance which could be due to the physical consequences of starvation.

Fourthly, if she was still unwilling to remain on the ward, I would make an application for her to be detained under section 3 of the 1983 Mental Health Act (it could prove necessary for the Responsible Medical Officer or his nominated deputy to carry out a section 5(2) to allow time for the section 3 assessment to be completed).

Fifthly, regardless of whether or not she was detained under the Mental Health Act, I would strive to obtain her agreement with her treatment plan.

The resolution of conflicts due to instrumental action, provocation, or personality factors is often successful with patience, and the skilled use of problem-solving techniques.

REFERENCES AND FURTHER READING

Bluglass RS. *A Guide to the Mental Health Act*. Edinburgh: Churchill Livingstone, 1983.

---

5 Under *common law*, the treatment of a voluntary patient requires his/her valid consent. He/she must have given consent freely (and without coercion) having understood the nature of the treatment and its likely effects. Doctors can only give treatment without such consent if it is crucial to protect the life and health of the patient.

Department of Health and the Welsh Office. *Code of Practice: Mental Health Act 1983*. London: HMSO, 1990.

Gelder M, Gath D, Mayou R. *Oxford Textbook of Psychiatry* (second edition). Oxford: Oxford University Press, 1989; Appendix p 897–903.

QUESTION 30C

You have been asked to see a 45 year old restaurant owner who was pressurised by his wife to seek medical help for his gambling problem. She is threatening to leave him because of mounting gambling debts, and he has borrowed heavily against his business to sustain his habit. He says he just needs to recover his losses, and then he will stop. He is restless and irritable when he is not able to gamble, and is only thrilled when the stakes are high.

What would the salient points of your assessment be?

What would your management be?

ANSWER 30C

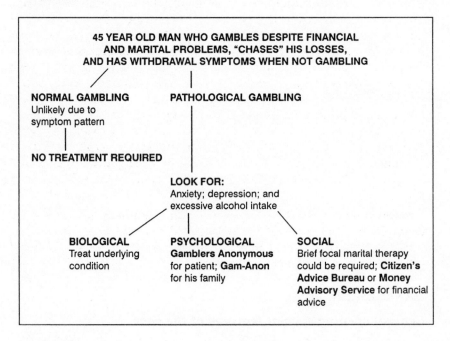

ASSESSMENT

General opening/special features of the case

His gambling is pathological[6] because it is characterised by: an inability to stop gambling despite mounting debts; restlessness and irritability when unable to gamble; "chasing" his losses; and his requirement to raise the stakes to achieve a thrill.

---

6   The South Oaks Gambling Screen is a useful method of quantifying the severity of gambling behaviour (a score of >5 suggests pathological gambling.)

Sources of history

I would interview the patient and his wife, separately at first, and then together.

History and mental state examination

Biological
I would look for a family history of mental illness, and a personal history of *anxiety, depression, excessive alcohol intake* and other *substance misuse disorders*.

Psychological
I would take a detailed history of the onset and progression of his gambling – when did he start gambling? Who encouraged or introduced him to gambling? Did he have a circle of gambling friends? Did he have an escalating pattern of gambling? When did he start gambling regularly? Did he have withdrawal symptoms when he was unable to gamble (irritability, restlessness and depression similar in nature to alcohol withdrawal symptoms are common)? What behaviours increase his risk of gambling (e.g. excessive alcohol consumption or dysthymia?); and *identify the "stages of change" of his behaviour* – Did he recognise any need to change his behaviour (*pre-contemplation*)? Did he acknowledge that he has a problem but is unwilling to change (*contemplation*)? Was he taking any steps (*action*) to change? Was he able to sustain (*maintenance*) not gambling?

Social
I would fully assess the *impact of his gambling on his family* – for example, what is the attitude of him and his wife to his marriage? What is the extent of his financial difficulties? Are there any legal proceedings for debts against him?

MANAGEMENT

General opening/special features of the case

The effectiveness of psychiatric treatment is uncertain.

Biological
Treat any underlying mental illness as appropriate.

Psychological
Self-help groups are the mainstay of treatment: he would be asked to contact *Gamblers Anonymous*,[7] who would move him along the *"stages of change"*,[8] and his family could be supported at *Gam-Anon*.

---

7 Treatment through *Gamblers Anonymous* has three stages: assessment, education about the addictive process and psychotherapy/counselling. Family education and support is usually carried out by *Gam-Anon*.

Social

Frequently, brief focal marital counselling sessions are also needed.

Financial advice should be sought from his local *Citizens Advice Bureau* or *Money Advice Service*.

REFERENCES AND FURTHER READING

Gelder M, Gath D, Mayou R. *Oxford Textbook of Psychiatry* (second edition). Oxford: Oxford University Press, 1989; chapter 22 p 889–90.

Lesieur HR, Blume SB. The South Oaks Gambling Screen (SOGS): a new instrument for the identification of pathological gamblers. *American Journal of Psychiatry 1988*; 144: 1184–8.

Orford J. Pathological gambling and its treatment. *British Medical Journal* 1988; 2296: 729–30.

Wray I. Cessation of high frequency gambling and withdrawal symptoms. *British Journal of Addiction* 1981; 76: 401–5.

Gambers Anonymous and *Gam-Anon*: 17/23 Blantyre Street, Chenys Walk, London SW10 0RP. Tel: 071-351-6794.

8 *Stages of change*" cross reference Question 27A.

CHAPTER 31

PARANOID STATE, MORBID JEALOUSY AND FOLIE À DEUX

QUESTION 31A

You have been asked to assess a 45 year old married man by his general practitioner, who believes his wife is being unfaithful and is demanding to know who it is so that he can face him "man to man".

ANSWER 31A

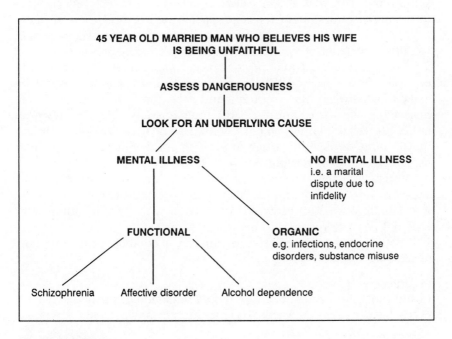

ASSESSMENT

General opening/special features of the case

The patient probably has *morbid jealousy*.

The two parts to his assessment would be the diagnosis of the underlying condition, and the evaluation of his *dangerousness*[1] to his wife, and other persons.

I would exercise great care to fully elicit his persecutory symptoms. This could prove difficult because he could: avoid the discussion; seek my collusion with his delusions; or react angrily when questioned.

Sources of history

I would interview his wife and himself separately at first, and then together.

History and mental state examination

Biological
I would look for a family or personal history of mental illness (especially of a *paranoid psychosis* or *alcohol dependence*).

I would assess the nature, onset and progression of the persecutory symptoms. The distinction between whether he believed he was deserving of punishment for some past action or had been unjustly wronged would differentiate between a *depressive* and a *paranoid condition*; evidence of *mood disorder, schizophrenia, excessive drinking* (by taking an alcohol history), or *organic impairment* (by testing his cognitive function) would be sought; and an association would be looked for between his symptoms and behaviour – how firmly did he believe his wife was unfaithful? How much hostility did he feel towards either his wife or her alleged paramour? Has he been cross-examining, questioning, or assaulting her, or seeking proof of her infidelity (such as semen stains in her pants)? If he has been plotting violence, was it towards himself, his wife, or others? What did he think might provoke the violence? Has he already been violent towards his wife, and if so, how was this provoked and how much injury did she suffer? How did his wife respond to his accusations?

I would also pay attention to any history of conflict in the marriage, or of sexual[2] difficulty.

Psychological
I would look for evidence of a *paranoid personality*, particularly with excessive sensitivity towards loss of status or self-esteem.

---

1 Morbid jealousy is a dangerous clinical condition; 12% of the men and 15% of the women in Broadmoor Hospital are there for this reason.

2 Repressed homosexuality by Freud, erectile impotence in men and sexual dysfunction in women (Vauhkonen K. on the pathogenesis of morbid jealousy. *Acta Psychiatrica Scandinavica 1968, supplement 202*), have, traditionally, been associated with morbid jealousy; more contemporary systematic evidence does not support this view).

Social
I would investigate the possibility of geographically separating the couple, at least until his symptoms have been brought under control.

REFERENCES AND FURTHER READING

Enoch MD, Trethowan WH. *Uncommon Psychiatric Syndromes* (second edition). Bristol: Wright, 1979.

Gelder M, Gath D, Mayou R. *Oxford Textbook of Psychiatry* (second edition). Oxford: Oxford University Press, 1989; chapter 10 p 334–7 and 341–2.

Shepherd M. Morbid jealousy: some clinical and social aspects of psychiatric symptoms. *Journal of Mental Science* 1961; 107: 687–753.

Soyka M, Naber G, Volcker A. Prevalence of delusional jealousy in psychiatric disorders: an analysis of 93 cases. *British Journal of Psychiatry* 1991; 158: 549–53.

QUESTION 31B

You have been asked to see a 65 year old woman who is complaining that her neighbour is conspiring to kill her because she has great powers. She has threatened to kill him first if she gets the chance. She has no past history of psychiatric illness.

What is the diagnosis?

Outline the principles of your management.

ANSWER 31B

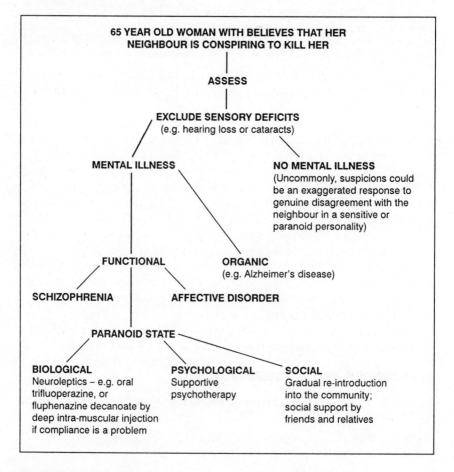

MAIN DIAGNOSIS

The most likely cause of the paranoid delusions would be a *paranoid state*.

General opening/special features of the case

The assessment[3] would be carried out in her home with the help of reliable informants.

PRINCIPLES OF MANAGEMENT

I would: *firstly*, look for evidence of a sensory deficit (e.g. hearing loss, or cataracts) which could exacerbate or produce paranoia.

Secondly, ascertain whether the paranoid beliefs could be due to an exaggerated but understandable response to genuine disagreements with the neighbours, the coarsening of a sensitive and insecure premorbid personality (*Der sensitive Beziehungswahn*), an organic condition (e.g. Alzheimer's disease), or a functional disorder such as *late onset schizophrenia* or *affective disorder*.

Thirdly, decide where treatment should take place – strong indicators of in-patient treatment include social disturbance or aggression towards the neighbours.

Fourthly, seek her voluntary admission, but if this was refused, apply for her detention under *Section 2 of the 1983 Mental Health Act* in the interests of her health and safety and to protect her neighbour from possible assault.

Fifthly, regardless of whether or not she was on a section, persuade her to take neuroleptic medication (e.g. *trifluoperazine*) voluntarily – suspicion about the purpose of the medication (some patients believe they are being poisoned) might be overcome by explaining that it would provide relief from troublesome symptoms such as sleeplessness and anxiety. If the medication was refused in tablet form, or compliance was a problem, it could be administered as a syrup; alternatively *fluphenazine decanoate* could be given by deep intramuscular injection.

Sixthly, provide *supportive psychotherapy*.

Finally, after she has recovered gradually introduce her back into the community by fostering the support of family and friends.

REFERENCES AND FURTHER READING

Enoch MD, Trethowan WH. *Uncommon Psychiatric Syndromes*. Bristol: Wright (1979).

Gelder M, Gath D, Mayou R. *Oxford Textbook of Psychiatry* (second edition). Oxford: Oxford University Press, 1989; chapter p 342–3.

Hirsch SR, Shepherd M. *Themes and Variations in European Psychiatry*. Bristol: John Wright, 1974.

Retterstol N. *Paranoia and Paranoid Psychoses*. Springfield, Il: CC Thomas, 1966.

---

3 Clinical guidelines for the assessment of paranoid patients have been discussed in Question 31A.

QUESTION 31C

You have been asked by a worried general practitioner to see two sisters in their 50's who have lived together for ten years in a remote part of the village because they are "sounding strange". They have not left the house for a couple of weeks, and have been barricading their windows. The general practitioner, who has spoken to both of them on the phone because they have refused to let him in, has informed you that their reason for barricading the windows was to protect themselves from evil people in the outside world. They have no close relatives.

What is the most likely diagnosis?

Outline how you would organise and arrange your assessment.

ANSWER 31C

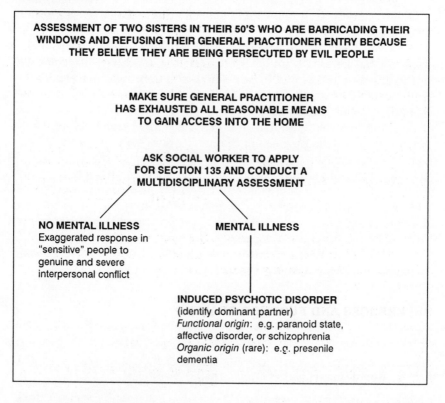

DIFFERENTIAL DIAGNOSIS

Induced psychotic disorder or *folie à deux* is a rare condition in which the dominant partner of a relationship (usually between two sisters) induces paranoid delusions, often after initial resistance, in the subordinate partner.

The differential diagnosis includes independent paranoid illnesses in both sisters, and an exaggerated response to severe interpersonal conflict in two sisters with extremely sensitive personalities.

OUTLINE OF THE ASSESSMENT

Medico-legal
I would: *firstly*, satisfy myself that the general practitioner had done all in his power to gain access into their home – including soliciting the help of someone with whom they had a favourable relationship.

Secondly, ask the *duty social worker* to apply for a warrant, from the magistrate's court (under *Section 135 of the 1983 Mental Health Act*), which would allow forcible access to the sisters' home, and their removal to a place of safety.

Thirdly, conduct the assessment[4] with the general practitioner, social worker, and a member of the community psychiatric team to identify the dominant[5] partner (who, usually, has a past psychiatric history, and more florid psychotic symptoms), make a diagnosis (e.g. *schizophrenia, affective disorder, paranoid state* or rarely, an *organic condition* such as presenile dementia) and plan treatment at the place of safety (i.e. hospital).

Psychological
Fourthly, arrange for the subordinate partner to be supervised and supported at home by the general practitioner and community psychiatric team, and *family therapy* could be indicated at a later date to establish a more equal relationship between the sisters.

Social
Finally, with the social worker, assess the subordinate partner's social needs in the community – examples include "meals on wheels", home help, or attendance at a day centre.

REFERENCES AND FURTHER READING

Cross reference question 31B: Enoch and Trethowan (1979).

Gelder M, Gath D, Mayou R. *Oxford Textbook of Psychiatry* (second edition). Oxford: Oxford University Press, 1989; chapter 10 p 340.

---

4 Clinical guidelines for the assessment of paranoid patients have been discussed in question 31A.
5 If the dominant partner was not readily identifiable, it would be prudent to admit both partners to separate wards for observation. With separation, the subordinate partner would be expected to rapidly relinquish her paranoid delusions.

CHAPTER 32

POST-TRAUMATIC STRESS DISORDER AND BATTLE SHOCK

QUESTION 32A

A 19 year old university student was involved in a train crash six months ago. His performance at university has started to deteriorate. And, he is complaining about having nightmares every night about trains crashing.

What would your management be?

ANSWER 32A

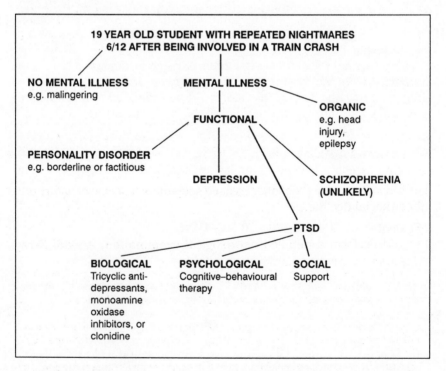

ASSESSMENT

General opening/special features of the case

Management is dependent on assessment.

The purpose of my assessment would be to find out whether his symptoms were due to *post-traumatic stress disorder (PTSD)*, injuries sustained (e.g. head injury) during the train crash, or some other mental disorder. It is also possible that he does not have a mental disorder.

Sources of history

I would wish to interview the patient, and any reliable informants. I would seek his permission to obtain any relevant medical or psychiatric records, and a progress report from his tutor.

History and mental state examination

Biological
I would look for a family or personal his.ory of mental illness or epilepsy. I would be interested in: the onset and progression of his symptoms (especially the three components[1] of PTSD), and evidence of a *depressive illness* or a *generalised anxiety state*. *Schizophrenia* would be a remote possibility.

Psychological
I would look for a history of *conduct disorder* and *traumatic events in childhood*, and carefully assess his *personality*.

I would explore the impact[2] of the symptoms on his life (e.g. does he currently avoid using trains?). If there was a history of head injury, I would arrange psychometric tests[3] to look for cognitive deficits.

Social
I would look for any proof of decreased sociability (e.g. *social withdrawal*), or social decline.

Physical
I would perform a detailed neurological examination. A skull X-ray

---

1 The three components of PTSD are: reliving of the stressor through nightmares and day dreams; emotional blunting, especially towards personal relationships; and associated symptoms of autonomic arousal (e.g. dysphoria, anxiety, hyperarousal, and cognitive deficits).

2 The impact of the event, and its likelihood of producing PTSD can be measured on the Impact of Event Scale (Horowitz et al. *Psychosomatic Medicine* 1979; 41: 209–18).

3 Social decline can be measured against the patient's own history (his tutor's report may comment on this), and the level of achievement of his parents. Progressive social decline can be associated with schizophrenia.

and an electroencephalogram would be carried out if he had sustained a head injury or there was a suspicion of epilepsy.

MANAGEMENT

General opening/special features of the case

The most likely diagnosis is PTSD.

My treatment would be aimed, at first, at providing symptomatic relief; secondly, at providing psychological support; and thirdly, at improving his performance at university and his social readjustment.

Biological

I would prescribe a sedative tricyclic *antidepressant* (e.g. trimi-pramine) to reduce arousal, to help with sleep, and to combat symptoms of dysphoria and anxiety which are common. *Monoamine oxidase inhibitors* and *clonidine* or *propranolol* are also possibilities. I would hesitate to use a benzodiazepine (and even then only in the short-term) because of the risk of dependence.

Psychological

I would encourage him to openly and freely discuss, review and re-live (using tapes) his traumatic experiences within a time-limited *cognitive-behavioural* framework.

Social

I would encourage him to seek support locally (i.e. from friends and relatives).

REFERENCES AND FURTHER READING

Burns TP, Hollins SC. Psychiatric response to the Clapham rail crash. *Journal of the Royal Society of Medicine* 1991; 84: 15–19.

Gelder M, Gath D, Mayou R. *Oxford Textbook of Psychiatry* (second edition). Oxford: Oxford University Press, 1989; Chapter 6 p 164 and 172.

Thompson GN. Post-traumatic psychoneurosis: evaluation of drug therapy. *Diseases of the Nervous System* 1977; 38: 617–9.

Van der Kolk BA, Van der Hart O. Pierre Janet and the breakdown of adaptation in psychological trauma. *American Journal of Psychiatry* 1989; 146(12): 1530–40.

QUESTION 32B

Your hospital, which is close to a war zone, has been designated to receive war casualties. One such casualty, a 22 year old man, was admitted with four of his comrades to the surgical ward, a day after being wounded in action. Although his wounds have been tended, and he appears to be physically comfortable, he has been unable to sleep. He has also been reported to spend most of his time "scanning" the ward environment, and to complain of tiredness.

How would you arrive at a differential diagnosis?

How would you manage the most likely disorder?

ANSWER 32B

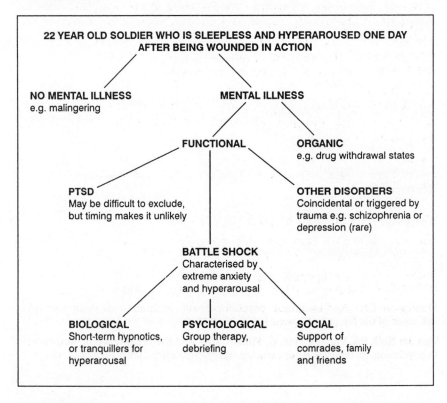

ASSESSMENT

General opening/special features of the case

To reach a differential diagnosis, I would need to assess him.

Sources of history

I would interview the patient himself, and his comrades.

History and mental state examination

Biological
I would look for any past, family or personal history of mental illness.

In his mental state, I would be interested in any evidence of *psychosis* (e.g. *schizophrenia*), *depression*, *hysteria*, *substance misuse*, or *PTSD*. And, I would also look for symptoms of extreme anxiety such as *hyperarousal*, *hypervigilance*, *dissociative symptoms* (e.g. sensorimotor or memory impairment) and *lassitude*.

Psychological
I would assess his personality, and explore any motives he may have for wishing to leave the army. I would like to know about the *dangerousness* of his posting, the *intensity of combat*, and how he came about his injury. I would look for any proof of *secondary gain*.

Social
I would assess the level of support from his comrades.

Physical examination
I would look for evidence that this may be a drug withdrawal state, especially from opiates (e.g. search for needle tracts or infections), and carry out a urine drug screen.
I would also review his surgical notes.

Differential diagnosis
See algorithm.

MANAGEMENT

General opening/special features of the case

The most likely diagnosis is *battle shock*.[4]

There are three general principles of management. They are:

(a) *immediacy* – treating the disorder as soon as possible to avoid chronicity;

(b) *proximity* – keeping the casualties as close to the combat zone as possible; and

(c) *expectancy* – providing comfort and rest.

---

4 Battle shock, a normal physiological reaction associated with intense combat, physical injury, and undertaking dangerous missions, is characterised by symptoms of overwhelming fear or anxiety such as hyperarousal and hyper-vigilance, and may include dissociative symptoms such as sensorimotor or memory impairment, or lassitude.
An interesting (but non-medical) book is *Catch 22* by Joseph Heller, published by Black Swan (1985).

Biological
I would only use a hypnotic, or a minor tranquilliser, for example a benzodiazepine, in the short-term (to avoid dependence).

Psychological
I would ensure that he is kept on the same ward as his comrades from the same regiment. Using a *Rogerian* approach, dealing with the "*here and now*", I would provide appropriate comforts and rest, and encourage him to talk openly and freely in a group with his comrades. I would ensure that there is *abreaction* of intense feelings such as fear, anger or helplessness. I would arrange a *debriefing* session on the fourth day, or as soon as possible thereafter.

Social
I would foster the support of comrades, and arrange for him to be re-introduced gradually to active duty.

REFERENCES AND FURTHER READING

Artiss KL. Human behaviour under stress – from combat to social psychiatry. *Military Medicine* 1963; 128: 1011–5.

Brandon S. The psychological aftermath of war. *British Medical Journal* 1991; 302: 305–6.

Johnson BA, Noble J. Helping the psychological victims of war. (In press, 1991).

Solomon Z, Benbenishty R, Mikulincer M. A follow-up of Israeli casualties of combat stress reaction ("battle shock") in the 1982 Lebanon War. *British Journal of Clinical Psychology* 1988; 27: 125–35.

MAIN INDEX

SUBJECT INDEX